Welcome

I'm glad that you have found this book. I sincerely hope that it can help make your life even a little bit easier.

For most people in pain, pain relief is the absolute top priority – and that is the main focus of this book. This book is about real and physical pain and the people who battle every day with this pain.

Long-term or chronic pain can also cause huge changes to a person's life, especially when physical injuries come on suddenly after car accidents, falls or accidents at work. Almost every part of a person's life can be affected: marriage and family, work, sleep, financial security and the everyday quality of life. This book is also devoted to helping people in pain rebuild their lives.

Ninety percent of my patients, over the past 20 plus years, have been people with chronic pain. My days are spent listening and learning from people in pain. This is where my best ideas come from. I like to share these ideas in the talks I give to community groups. If you send an email to me, I will make sure to send you a copy of one of my most popular talks.

Thank you.

Yours with care,

Michael R. MacDonald, Ph.D.

Please go to my website www.UnbelievablePainControl.com click on the link for a Free Booklet and request a copy of: *A Simple Survival Guide for Chronic Pain and Fibromyalgia.*

Unbelievable PAIN CONTROL

How to Heal and Recover from Chronic Pain and Fibromyalgia

Michael R. MacDonald, Ph.D.

Michael Renford Books

Library and Archives Canada Cataloguing in Publication

MacDonald, M. R., 1954 -
Unbelievable pain control : How to heal and recover from
chronic pain and fibromyalgia / Michael R. MacDonald.

Includes bibliographical references and index.
ISBN 978-0-9812078-0-3

1. Chronic pain–Treatment–Popular works.
2. Fibromyalgia–Treatment–Popular works. I. Title.

RB127.M328 2009 616'.0472 C2009-900995-1

PUBLISHER:
Michael Renford Books
655 Wellington Road South, Suite 401
London, Ontario N6C 4R4
www.renfordbooks.com
www.UnbelievablePainControl.com

EDITING AND PROJECT MANAGEMENT:
Debbie Elicksen, Nancy Syrett,
Freelance Communications, Calgary, Alberta

DESIGN AND PRODUCTION:
Tammy Golinski, Kervyn Corporation, London, Ontario

PRINTING:
Friesens, Altona, Manitoba

Unbelievable Pain Control: How to Heal and Recover from Chronic Pain and Fibromyalgia – First Edition
Printed and Bound in Canada
Copyright 2009

Important Note: This book was written to provide general information about various types of chronic pain, including fibromyalgia. It is published with the understanding that the author and publisher are not offering psychological or medical advice to readers. It is not intended for readers to assume that the ideas contained here should replace any advice or treatments from their psychologists, physicians, therapists, or lawyers. Readers should consult their health care providers regarding the care and treatment of any health problems. Readers should consult their lawyers for advice regarding any legal, insurance or workers' compensation matters.

For Susie and Kaylie,
I love you.

Acknowledgments

Thank you to the many people who have helped and believed in me, over all of these years. Thank you Susie, I love you and feel very fortunate to have been able to share my life with you. Your compassion and dedication to everyone you care about amazes me every day. You and Kaylie are my life. Thank you Kaylie, our bundle of joy from day one. I love you and am very proud of you.

I feel blessed to have been surrounded by a loving family, who always believed in me. Thank you Mom and Dad, Jeff and Alyson. You are always with me. A second loving family came along when I married Susie. Thank you for all of your kindness and support – Ruth and Garry, Rob and Eleanor, Scott, Cathy and Randy. I know I can always count on you. A dear group of friends has been with me since grade two. That's amazing. We don't see each other as often as we should. Thank you Jerry, John and Jeff. You are an inspiration.

In my professional life, I have been helped by truly inspiring mentors. Thank you Lester Krames, Nick Kuiper, Warren Nielson, Gail Golden and Barry Death. You have given much of yourselves. I am very grateful and honored. I am also very fortunate to have worked with many talented colleagues. We cannot do this kind of work alone, trying to find new and better ways of helping people in pain, year after year. Thank you Robert Schnurr,

Owen Garrett, Gani Braimoh, Peter Pryor, Jeff McKillop, Ann McDermid, Shannon Stewart, Wendy Lewis, Michelle Duwyn, Charles Nelson, Jeni Gagne and Lisa Lee. I appreciate your big hearts and your devotion to this important work. Also, a special thank you to the many patients we have had the privilege to work with, over the past 20 plus years. Learning from you, hour by hour, day by day, has made a real difference.

Thank you with all my heart.

Author's Note

All of the characters that appear in Book One and Book Two, Part One are fictional. The characters Suzanne, Ashley, Sarah and Mike also appear periodically throughout all three books. They do not represent any specific individuals or patients known to Dr. MacDonald. Any similarities are coincidental. Suzanne is a fictional character introduced in Book One. Her experiences of having surgery without anesthesia have been inspired by the real life experiences of Dr. Victor Rausch. This is explained in Book Two, Part Two. His amazing accomplishments have been well documented and referenced.

Most of the sections in this book have been written for the benefit of all readers. Some parts are more technical. The more scientific aspects may be beyond some readers. Yet, I felt that even a basic awareness of the amazing work that is being done all around the world might provide some much needed hope for people in pain.

Book Three reviews work done by many incredible organizations. These organizations and societies are devoted to helping the millions of people throughout the world who live in pain. This information is readily available from the Websites I referenced. These Websites are constantly being updated. Please search out each Website to find out about their most current work.

Thank you and welcome to ***Unbelievable Pain Control.***

Table of Contents

General Introduction

Experts ranged in serried rows
Fill the enormous plaza full;
But only one is there who knows,
And he's the one who fights the bull.

– Robert Graves –

And he's the one who lives the pain.

It is not easy coming to see a psychologist when you have physical injuries and pain. You don't know what to expect. You may not even know why you were referred to us in the first place. To help you feel comfortable, I usually start by describing the kind of work I do.

First, I explain that if you have short-term pain, you would never end up coming to see a psychologist like me. If your pain settles down within a few months, you can return to your normal life. This situation is not so hard to manage. Not much stress is involved.

If your pain and injuries continue, month after month, then your life starts to unravel. Stresses and forced life changes start to build. Maybe you have been unable to work because of painful injuries and are uncertain when or if you can ever work again. You may have trouble getting income replacement benefits. Your pain and limitations may disrupt family life: your spouse and children may become overwhelmed with the extra load on them. Worst of all, the stress caused by your injuries and limitations may be wearing you down, making you irritable, interfering with your sleep and making it harder for you to cope with your never-ending pain. At this point, you don't even know where to start getting your pain and your life back under control. Prolonged stressful situations like this are hard for anyone to manage. This is where I can help.

My life has been dedicated to helping people in pain heal and recover. My goal is to reduce the enormous suffering that comes with chronic pain and fibromyalgia and to help people rebuild their lives. Ninety percent of my patients, over the past 20 plus years, are individuals who live each day in pain. My days are spent listening and learning. I get to spend a lot of time with each person. In this way, I can really get to know their injuries, their pain and how it has affected their lives.

Chronic pain is real and physical pain. It affects well over ten percent of the population. Millions of people live every day in pain. Chronic pain is a leading cause of disability and work loss. It is never 'all in your head'. It can be caused by any type of painful injury or illness. Neck and back injuries, headaches and fibromyalgia are among the most common types of chronic pain. Sometimes, chronic pain can follow from repetitive or traumatic work injuries, injuries from car accidents or illnesses like arthritis. So what has psychology got to do with it?

It is true that chronic pain is not a psychological injury or illness. Chronic pain is a legitimate, physical problem. But, chronic pain is more than just pain. At its core, chronic pain is long-term pain. Day after day, month after month, the disruption to your life builds, when your pain never lets up. It can seep into every corner of your life. Your stress levels rise. In turn, these high stress levels can aggravate your physical injuries and pain, just like stress can aggravate any medical health problem. Pain and high stress levels create further problems, such as poor sleep, emotional difficulties, and strains in relationships with your family. Relentless pain is the cause of these additional problems, which then interfere with your ability to cope with the pain itself. It becomes a vicious cycle – pain causes stress, which leads to more pain, then more stress, creating bigger and bigger problems in your life. This is part of what makes chronic pain so complicated – and overwhelming for so many people.

If you live in pain, or know someone that does, you know that nothing is more important than pain relief – or better yet, a cure if possible. But traditional medicine can only do so much. Unfortunately, many painful injuries and illnesses have no cure – yet. If you live in pain, you know that long-term pain can lead to serious losses. Almost every part of your life can be affected: marriage, family, work, sleep, financial security, your emotions and the everyday quality of your life. These losses (and stresses) can aggravate your physical injuries and lead to more pain, more limitations and even greater losses. This is a very difficult pattern to reverse.

I wrote this book to help you lessen your pain, to help you reduce your losses and to help you rebuild your life. I believe that all of these parts are important. As you will see throughout this book, a focus on these three goals will provide you with your best chance of long-term pain control. I sincerely hope that this book can help make your life even a little easier. Below is a brief summary.

• • •

This book, *Unbelievable Pain Control*, is organized in an unusual way. It is set up like three books in one. Each book has a different format, tone and set of ideas. Some books are more focused on methods for healing and recovery, although with different formats. Another book is more technical with a large reference section. I have created a detailed Table of Contents to help you find your way to the parts of the book that can help you the most. Below is a breakdown of what is in each book.

Book One is a fictional story based on a true and unbelievable event. It tells the amazing story of a dentist, who willingly undergoes major surgery without anesthesia. Three patients who have been admitted to a chronic pain program hear about this story. They are overwhelmed at first, and not sure what to make of an individual that undergoes surgery this way. All three patients are not even sure of the possibility that an individual could have such control over pain. They themselves have been struggling and overwhelmed with their own pain. As chance would have it, they get to meet this fellow patient and learn more details about how she was able to achieve such unbelievable pain control. As they get to know each other, she agrees to teach them methods of pain control that help them with their own painful injuries.

In Book One you meet Ashley. She is one of the four patients in the hospital pain program. She is a very diligent note taker. Based on Ashley's notes, Book Two reveals the ideas and methods that each patient learned from their doctors, and from each other, as they progressed through the hospital chronic pain program. Simple ideas about pain control, healing and recovery are explained in this book. In Book Two you will also learn about Dr. Victor Rausch. He is the real deal and the inspiration behind Suzanne, the character in Book One who underwent surgery without anesthesia. I had the opportunity to meet Dr. Rausch many years ago. He is even more interesting and impressive in person.

Book Three introduces you to many of the incredible organizations around the world that are devoted to helping people in pain. You will meet some of today's top doctors and scientists. Two doctors in particular have personal, as well as professional expertise in chronic pain. We can all learn a lot from their work and their writings. Book Three also includes details about the largest scientific investigation of chronic pain ever done.

This is an exciting time in the field of chronic pain. So much is being learned. So much is being done. The reality of chronic pain as a serious and legitimate health problem is no longer in doubt. Hopefully the dark days of denial are behind us at last. The Epilogue takes you on a tour of just how far scientists have progressed. Top doctors in this field help you to see the many new discoveries on the horizon. Hope is often in short supply when lives are filled with pain. In this last section, and throughout this book, I have tried to be realistic yet hopeful. The long-term relief of pain is a vital goal, for the individuals and families that suffer, and for our progress toward a decent and caring society.

One of my favorite quotes is by Bill Moyers from his book, *Healing and the Mind (1993, p.26):*

"Caring is good medicine"

Another one of my favorite quotes is inscribed on a small plaque in my office:

"Kindness is Power"

Book One

UNBELIEVABLE PAIN CONTROL

Often, when I try to help individuals in pain, I use stories and examples. It is easier, sometimes, to get an idea across when it is embedded in a relevant and interesting tale. People like to hear about others' experiences, whether they be struggles or triumphs. We often learn best by following the paths that others have laid before us. Professionals, as well, can often learn best with case studies and detailed examples.

What follows is a fictional story. It is inspired by an amazing true event - an unbelievable accomplishment. (More about this real-life feat in Book Two). Yet, all the characters are purely fictional.

Suzanne is the main character of this story. It is her voice. Sometimes, she is philosophical like at the start of Book One. Other times, it is her struggles that takeover. I hope you can learn from Suzanne's story – learn about the realities of chronic pain and fibromyalgia, its impact on people's lives and the many paths to believable and unbelievable pain control. Hers is a story of hope, healing and recovery.

At the end of Book One, I have included a Notes section where you can find detailed information about chronic pain and fibromyalgia. This section, based on scientific studies, gives you an overview of the symptom patterns, causes, and incidence of chronic pain and fibromyalgia around the world.

CHAPTER ONE

Hope and Possibility

When you are healthy, everything is possible. You have the energy to do whatever you want, whenever you want. Serious illness can happen, of course, but rarely, and only to other people. If you do get sick, you can fight it off and be back on your feet in no time. Many people are lucky to be able to think like this. I know I was.

Life does not feel this way, though, when pain, injury, or illness strikes – if you are knocked down suddenly, a blow from out of nowhere. Or when it lasts. Pain and stress can wear you down more than you had ever thought possible. When pain has no end in sight, you struggle to find even the faintest light. You keep searching for signs of hope – some offer of relief, some cure, or some path that will bring you back to your normal life. You want to hope, to believe in possibilities again.

• • •

There was a time when I had lost almost all hope. I had been living in pain, hour-by-hour, for over two years. This was serious pain. Aching, burning, relentless pain that kept me up at night and limited almost everything I tried to do. I could not see my way to the next day, let alone to the possibility of a future without pain. My well-grounded husband could see a way for me, though – even a return to my former self. I thought he was delusional.

He encouraged me to enter a program to help people with long-term pain. This was a comprehensive pain program affiliated with the university. I would be admitted to hospital, stay there for six weeks, and have all my injuries fully investigated and treated. Medical specialists, nurses, and a full team of therapists and counselors would be there to help me. My husband and I both knew that there was no instant cure for my neck and back pain. But, I agreed to go anyway. Maybe something could be done.

CHAPTER TWO

The Chronic Pain Program

I stepped inside the door. It hit me: the institutional green paint, the odor of disinfectant, the people lined up along the hall asleep in their wheelchairs. I wanted to bolt for the door right then and there. Somehow, I kept walking.

The chronic pain program was in the physical medicine and rehabilitation department, up on the second floor. In the elevator were more old and frail people. They lived here on the first, third, and fourth floors of this hospital. My heart sank as I wondered whether this was really the right place for me.

At the second floor, the elevator opened to more green walls and worn out furniture, yet the feel of this space was different. It was full of life. The ward clerk welcomed me with a big smile. After a few simple questions, she escorted me down the hall to my room. My roommate, Ashley, was busy putting away her stuff: delicate print dresses, conservative, yet fashionable shoes, and a very pretty makeup bag. I felt like a leftover from the seventies with my faded jeans and baggy tops.

Ashley kept talking as I unpacked. She was younger than I was; late twenties, I guessed, to my mid-forties, with a bright and engaging manner. Ashley had already met Sarah and Mike, the other two patients in this pain program.

"Mike is this huge, friendly guy," she said. "He told me to call him Bear. I told him that I would stick with Mike, if that was okay with him."

I learned from Ashley that she was hoping for a near miracle to happen in our six-week program. She had been suffering from neck and right arm pain for the past three years, caused by having rolled her car off of an icy road. Over time, her neck and arm pain escalated. She was only able to get about three to four hours of sleep on most nights. Finally, one specialist figured out that she had developed fibromyalgia, an illness that can follow from car accidents, prolonged neck pain and sleep deprivation. This diagnosis helped to explain her new symptoms of widespread body pain, irritable bowels, headaches, fatigue, and forgetfulness. Ashley had not given up hope, though. In her own quiet way, she persevered. She clung onto her faith that life had to get better, somehow.

I told Ashley that I, too, suffered from neck pain, as well as back pain and headaches. My injuries started suddenly after a fall outside my dental office. It was an icy day, and before I knew it, my feet were out from under me and I was flat on my back. That was twenty-six months ago and there had been little improvement. I leaned heavily on my husband during those months. He was a godsend. My hopes had been built up and crushed many times since my fall. This time I was determined to keep my hopes and feelings in check, or so I thought.

Later, at dinner, I learned Mike and Sarah had similar stories. Mike fell off of a scaffold at work and hurt his right shoulder. A drunk driver hit Sarah in her car, leaving her with severe back and leg pain. Together, we represented part of the ten to fifteen percent of the population that live in pain – constant pain, every day and night, week after week, year after year. We were burned out from sleepless nights, pain medication, physical limitations, financial losses, and wars with lawyers and insurance companies. This program was reserved for the worst cases of chronic pain. Sadly, we represented the worst of the worst.

Her years of torment were obvious from my first encounter with Sarah. She was pleasant, but guarded. There was an edge to her voice whenever any of us tried to be hopeful. She did not want to be in this program. Her specialist had recommended inpatient treatment. Then her lawyer told her that it would look bad for her lawsuit if she refused. Sarah felt trapped, with little choice, no control. To make matters worse, her three young children had to stay with her complaining mother for the six weeks she was in hospital.

In a funny way, Mike and Sarah looked like they could be brother and sister. Both were fairly large people, solid with short-cropped hair. They dressed in comfortable clothes. There were no pretensions about either of them.

In other ways, they were very different. There was no edge to Mike. He was fun to be around, a bit shy, but naturally open to people and new experiences. It was hard not to like such a warm and simple guy. He had suffered like the rest of us. For him, it was his aching right shoulder, the loss of his construction work, and many battles with the workers' compensation system. He was more than willing to give this program a try, though. We were all glad he was there to help liven up the place.

The first week was torture. We were bombarded with physiotherapy, occupational therapy, psychology, social work, recreational therapy, and even visits from a pastoral care counselor. We felt close to death on some days and joked that the pastor should just come in and read us our last rites.

Not one of us was able to go home that first weekend. We were hurting badly. I think Mike and Sarah were in the worst shape. They were weaned off all their pain medications. Their pain was heightened without the medication and they tried to fight off the irritability, nausea, and crawling-skin sensations that come with drug withdrawal. It was hell for them.

It was eleven o'clock on the Saturday night. No one could sleep, so we piled into Mike's room to keep each other company. We were all struggling and looking for some kind of sign that we would be able to endure this program and get some benefit from it. Hope seemed in short supply.

Sarah was particularly upset at John, the physiotherapist. He seemed to come from the boot camp school of therapy and was making enemies of us all. Sarah led us toward a night of endless complaining. I knew something had to be done or else we would all drown in our own despair.

I piped up and told the group about Cynthia, a rehab counselor I was working with over the past year. Cynthia was kind, full of hope, and kept her patients going with fascinating stories. I asked the group if they were up for an amazing tale. I knew from their faces that it was just what they needed.

CHAPTER THREE

An Amazing Story

One of Cynthia's best stories was about Suzanne.

Suzanne was a dentist and knew a lot about pain. She knew a needle full of freezing was the easiest way to get rid of the pain from drilling and cutting. Her patients didn't really like the needles, the freezing, or the lingering numbness and drooling. Who would? Suzanne wondered if she could find another method of pain control – maybe even a natural one.

This possibility intrigued Suzanne and she couldn't let it go. Her most difficult patient, a high-strung man who needed several cavities filled, spurred her on one day. He started to wind himself up in the dental chair, before Suzanne had even touched him. Then he sprung into a full panic, just seeing the stainless steel needle full of freezing coming toward him. He bolted from the chair, sending her tray of instruments spinning across the floor. Two of Suzanne's assistants rushed in to help. It took more than twenty minutes before they could calm the man down. Finally, he allowed Suzanne to inject him with the freezing. Ninety minutes later, they were done. Suzanne was exhausted. There must be a better way, she thought, I never want to go through this again.

Suzanne went to the university library that next Sunday afternoon. She started researching how people coped with pain in the days before freezing was invented. During one of her searches, she discovered that painful dental procedures and even surgeries had often been performed without pain medication. She learned about a famous English surgeon working in India, who had used hypnosis to help his patients manage their pain during surgery. Dr. James Esdaile performed over one thousand such operations in the 1800s.

Suzanne was intrigued by this research. It made sense to her. She had had some experience with hypnosis and relaxation training in dental school. One of her fellow students had taken a keen interest and liked to practice his new techniques on Suzanne and her friends. Suzanne was very curious about it, and liked exploring the different feelings she experienced while under hypnosis.

She never felt any loss of control like some people found. In fact, she felt more control, but in a relaxed, non-forced way. She learned new skills, with her regular practice, that she could use to reduce tension, school stresses, and even pain during the birth of her first child. These memories flooded back to her in the library, as she read through the hypnosis research and the incredible stories of surgery without anesthesia.

Suzanne was to have her gallbladder removed in the upcoming months. She knew it would be a painful, yet routine, surgical procedure. *Maybe, I could have it done without an anesthetic.* It was a crazy thought, but the possibility had taken root. Such operations had been done before with the assistance of a clinical hypnotist or acupuncturist. Never before, though, had an individual done such a thing on her own. Now, the idea became even more enticing. *I could make history.*

To start, Suzanne needed to figure out what she was up against. She had many questions, of course, and needed to know exactly what to expect. How long was the surgery going to take? What would the surgeon actually be doing after she was cut open? What parts of the surgery would be the most painful? How long would it take to recover? What would happen if she couldn't take the pain? Would there be an anesthetic available to her, just in case?

Suzanne's medical friend put her in touch with a surgeon she knew, Dr. Grace. They met in his office. Suzanne was brimming with nervous energy and had a million questions for him. He liked her spirit and agreed to help. If Suzanne could pull this off, he would like to be a part of it.

Dr. Grace provided useful details about the mechanics and step-by-step procedures involved. Suzanne always found the technical details interesting. This information helped Suzanne settle on her decision to go ahead. His confidence in her also helped to lessen some of her fear. Then, Dr. Grace and Suzanne went about preparing for the upcoming operation and rehearsed each step of each procedure.

This preparation was an important part of the pain control process. As a dentist, Suzanne knew that the more frightened patients became, the less able they were to control their pain. Fear causes alarm and makes you want to run, just like the panicked patient who almost ruined her dental office. What Suzanne needed was concentration and composure. This was the path to control. She knew she had to prepare to deal with her fear, just like she had to prepare to manage the pain.

The night before surgery was her first true test. Suzanne wondered if she would be able to sleep, knowing what lay ahead. And without a proper sleep, would she have the concentration and stamina to go through with the operation and the recovery?

Lying there in bed, she started calming herself by listening to taped sounds from the rainforest. This tape was one of her favorites. Then, she moved to a deeper state of relaxation with a technique called progressive relaxation. This procedure is a type of relaxation where you concentrate on tensing, then relaxing, each area of your body. You do this very slowly, allowing all your muscles to settle down, to feel loose, warm, and comfortable. The most important part of this technique is to identify what true relaxation feels like – in your mind and in each part of your body. Then, with practice, you can bring it on fast and deep. As Suzanne worked through her steps, she re-created that familiar bodily feeling. She was a blob of inner calm, no tension, like Jell-O plopped on the bed.

Next, while still relaxed, Suzanne turned to an imagination exercise she had been practicing. This exercise was like a dress rehearsal for the next day's big event. She pictured herself on a movie screen with Dr. Grace going through each surgical step on her body. She saw him do each part perfectly, a consummate professional. Suzanne felt connected with Dr. Grace's kindness and absolute confidence. He would take good care of her. She became absorbed in this drama, then drifted into a deep sleep.

The next morning, Suzanne awoke feeling refreshed and calm. She found no hints of any fear or indecision. A sense of inner peace had carried over from the night before. It had a dream-like quality. She knew what lay ahead, accepted it, and was ready for surgery.

They wheeled Suzanne into the operating room. She climbed up onto to the surgical table. She was given no medication – no pre-operative sedative, no pills, no anesthesia. Suzanne was calm and composed. There was a small audience around her, talking softly and not sure of what to expect. They never saw (or even heard of) anything like this before.

A needle was inserted into Suzanne's arm. The anesthetist did not give her medication or anesthesia, but was set-up in case of any emergency. Her pulse and blood pressure were monitored. Throughout the whole procedure, he kept a careful watch.

Before the first big cut, Suzanne readied herself with another technique she had been practicing. This involved a type of imaginary journey that would capture her attention and take her mind away from the pain of surgery. In the weeks before, she had put together an album of her favorite pictures. These included photos of her daughter and husband from the first years of her daughter's life. Each picture was chosen to bring back vivid memories of a time in her life that was filled with joy. She had discussed this strategy with Dr. Grace beforehand. If she should happen to smile during the operation, Suzanne wanted him to know that this was all part of her plan.

As Suzanne lay on the surgical table, she imagined herself on a sun-filled afternoon, settling into her favorite chair on her cottage porch. With cushions all around her, she started to leaf through her album of treasures. The first photo triggered warm and funny thoughts of her daughter's second birthday party. She allowed these memories to expand, bringing back the squeals of delight, the sights of children running around, the smell of birthday cake and candles. She could see the children's faces and feel their excitement. These fine details filled her senses.

Then she opened her eyes slightly, and smiled at Dr. Grace. He met her glance and knew she was ready. He felt along the line where the incision would be. Then he placed the scalpel on her belly and began several inches of cutting. Her blood pressure spiked immediately, from one hundred thirty-five to one hundred ninety. Her pulse rate jumped from eighty-two to one hundred fifteen beats per minute. It then took several minutes before her vital signs settled into a normal pattern.

During these first minutes, Suzanne felt a flowing sensation run through her entire body. This was an odd and interesting feeling that was hard to describe. Then her eyes opened and she found herself acutely aware of everything near her. She looked around briefly, noticing various items in the room, the people, and the novel sensations in her body. This heightened awareness did not scare her, nor did the pool of blood around the large incision. She did not flinch nor tense up. Her breathing stayed slow and deep. She knew that awareness was a necessary part of pain control.

Suzanne let her eyes rest again and returned to her memories. She could feel and hear her daughter's birthday party going on in her mind. Her dissociation was working, but not quite the way she had planned. She was in a state of deep relaxation and was feeling no pain. But she sensed that it would be difficult to stay this calm if she did not keep track of what was happening in the operation. Some anxiety, related to not knowing, might appear and undermine her concentration and control. She became aware that she needed to do something different, but didn't know exactly what.

It became a temptation to return to her memories and completely block out the physical sensations of being cut and probed during the surgery. This strategy had been working well so far. If she wanted, she could go into a deep and prolonged daydream, and wait for the operation to be over. This plan was dangerous, though. How could she have any real control over her body, by staying in the dark? Control needed to come with awareness, not with avoidance. Maybe there was some middle ground, she thought. Control is not something that is either black or white, on or off. It is the gray areas, in between, where real control happens.

Suzanne let herself come up to a lighter state of calm. Then, with some gentle direction, she flowed back into a deep state of relaxation. In this way, she could guide herself to the surface, check out what was happening in the operation, and then flow back into her deep state among the pictures and memories. She could allow herself to feel the sensations of being pulled and prodded by the surgeon, yet direct the flow of her attention away from any sensations of pain. This delicate balance, between dissociation and awareness, gave her the control she needed.

Suzanne felt completely detached from the sensations of pain. It was like being an observer, watching the operation happen. She was able to hear the team talking and joking. She could see their every move. Then, out of nowhere, came the realization that all this had happened in the first few minutes of the seventy-five minute operation. This was truly amazing.

Throughout the procedure, she perspired heavily. Yet, after their initial rise, both her pulse and blood pressure dropped to a normal level and held steady. From time to time, Suzanne would open her eyes, look at Dr. Grace and allow a faint smile. She would immediately feel stronger with this connection, her sense of control renewed.

The time passed quickly, and soon the final sutures were in place. Dr. Grace smiled at Suzanne, then asked if she was ready to walk back to her room. She climbed off the operating table, limped briefly back and forth, then clutching his arm, made it back to the elevator and down to her room.

This all happened on a Friday morning. The surgery took one hour and fifteen minutes. Suzanne was kept in hospital until the following Wednesday. This was back in 1990, when patients were kept in hospitals for almost a week following major surgery. Suzanne was discharged from the hospital on that Wednesday and returned to her dental office the following Monday, still without any medication.

CHAPTER FOUR

Was it a Dream?

Half an hour or so passed by the time I finished my story. Ashley, Sarah, and Mike were quiet. They seemed confused, not knowing what to make of what they had just heard. Mike was the first to break the silence.

"What a story. Can you imagine if such a thing were really possible? We wouldn't need to be stuck in a place like this."

"You're dreaming," answered Sarah. "We're in a place like this because such things are not possible. Maybe some guru on some mountain somewhere could do it, but not any kind of normal person."

Sarah paused for a moment, then continued her rapid speech. "You know, it really pisses me off to hear this. People are always giving us this crap that we should be trying harder. If we were really motivated, they say, we could overcome these pains and get back to work. Yeah right! This story would be great ammunition for my husband. He thinks like that. He doesn't even believe I'm in pain."

"But, what if it's true?" asked Mike. "We never really know, do we? Maybe, we all have some secret powers inside of us that we don't know how to use." The fantasy of having superpowers intrigued Mike since he was a young child. He still liked reading about comic book heroes, though he wouldn't admit to it.

Sarah stood up and stared right at him. "C'mon, Mike. If my insurance company ever heard of such a thing, they'd be all over me even more. My adjuster is always sending rehab workers around to push every new thing on me. If such things were possible, I would have heard about it, believe me." These kinds of stresses really got Sarah overheated.

"Mike," said Ashley, "it does seem kind of 'out there.' We've all been to see so many doctors. They have never told me about anything like that – not even close."

"Maybe not," I replied. "Sometimes, doctors avoid achievements like Suzanne's because they seem so extreme. Doctors don't know what to make of such things. They don't know how they work, so they are reluctant to tell their patients about them. Doctors are afraid of false hope. They know it will come back on them if things don't work out."

I paused, then went on slowly. "I am pretty sure this story is true. I know first hand – for real. I was there, under the knife. Me."

"What?" snapped Sarah.

Mike was still and trying to absorb what he had just heard.

"What did you just say?" asked Sarah.

"Yes, it's true. Me. I did it. I swear."

"I must be dreaming," said Ashley. "You did that? You can do such things? But, how?"

Mike piped up. “You have a lot of explaining to do, Suzanne.”

“I know I do. But, before you hit me with all your questions, let me fill in some missing details. I am a dentist; that’s right. Or at least I was until my fall that icy day. Now, I’m not so sure. The surgery did happen – it was major abdominal surgery, back when full incisions were made for this type of operation. Now, small little incisions are used, making it easier and less painful.”

They were still staring at me. “All the parts of the story are true, I swear.”

“You must admit, it was a pretty detailed story. I couldn’t make up a story like that. The operation was videotaped, written up in a scientific journal, and discussed at many conferences. Maybe, some of the doctors here in the pain clinic have heard or read about it.

“It was a big deal for me. Others have had even more painful procedures done without anesthetic. The medical history books are full of such stories. I had one important advantage over other patients, though. I had a choice. At any moment, I could have asked the doctor to knock me out, or add some pain or tranquilizing medication to the needle in my hand. With this choice, I had some extra control over the situation.”

Ashley and Mike sat quietly. Sarah was restless but not talking. They hadn’t stopped staring at me.

Then Sarah broke the silence in her usual blunt manner. “Forgive me, but I have to know. Why are you here, Suzanne – in this program? If you have such power, or control – or whatever – how come you don't just use it to heal yourself?"

Ashley and Mike perked up. They had been thinking about asking this same question.

I was taken aback by Sarah's directness. Then I gathered my thoughts and carried on. "I'm not sure I know the answer, Sarah. But let me try to answer. After my fall, I was pretty banged up and hurting a lot. I tried to convince myself that I would get better. I only needed a little time, I thought. I did use some of these techniques, then, to help with my pain and to keep going. I was starting to feel better. It was very slow, but improvement was happening."

Mike jumped in. "So what happened then?"

"Well, things started to change on me. Things fell apart – I fell apart. I began to lose control over everything: my pain, my work, my life. At least that's what it seems like as I look back.

"Six months after my accident, I was still not getting any better and was not any closer to being able to work. I was getting benefits from my insurance company. Then the adjuster sent me to one of their doctors. She did a brief examination, and sent a report to the insurance company saying that my injuries had healed and that there was no reason for me to be experiencing ongoing pain. My benefits were cut off after that. Then my life really started to spin out of control."

"This part I can believe," said Sarah. We all nodded in agreement.

"I had no income. This went on for months. My debts started piling up. My neck pain went way out of control. I had severe headaches all day long. My husband and children didn't understand what was happening, and didn't know how to help. The stress on all of us was unbearable. I sunk into a deep depression and eventually ended up here."

"This story just keeps getting more complicated," said Ashley. "What happened to the Suzanne who could control pain? Where did she go?"

"I got burned out, I think – all used up. I didn't want to give in. I was still trying, even nine or ten months after my fall. Month after month, though, my strength kept slipping away.

"Then, I lost my dental practice. And I was afraid of losing my family. The stress sent my neck and head pain soaring. My doctors couldn't help. I was so depressed that I didn't have the power to get out of bed some days. I felt like I had no control at all in my life. I just couldn't do it."

Sarah was getting impatient, listening to me go on and on. "Control over your life? What has that got to do with anything? Your pain wasn't caused by losing your life or your work."

"No, Sarah, it wasn't. My pain was caused by my fall. The loss of my dental practice came afterward."

"That's what I thought," followed Sarah. "I lost my marriage after my pain got so bad my husband couldn't take it or me any longer. But, my marriage didn't cause my pain. It didn't have anything to do with it. It's not why I am here."

"But, Sarah," said Mike, trying to diffuse the tension. "The breakdown of your marriage must have been a big stress for you. Wasn't it hard? Didn't it make you worse?"

"Yes it did," answered Sarah. "Much worse. But, so what?"

Ashley waded in. "Haven't we all been told, over and over again, that stress can make us worse? My doctors keep telling me to reduce the stresses in my life. They say that can help lessen my neck and arm pain and settle my fibromyalgia down."

"Yeah, yeah," said Sarah. I know. All this extra pain and stress makes me so angry, though – even more than my ex-husband. When I get angry, I make myself get going and do things. Too many things. This causes even more pain. It just keeps getting stronger while I get weaker."

"I got weaker, too," I said, "and started to wither. Without work, I had no money coming in. That was one big stress. And then when my insurance company cut my benefits, everything got even worse. I couldn't take how severe my headaches became. My back didn't flare up as much, but my neck pain and headaches were killing me."

"Okay, so all that stress made your pain worse. And these were big stresses. I can buy that," said Ashley.

"Yes," I explained. "It seemed that the stress and the higher pain levels knocked me down hard. It kicked the wind right out of me. It changed me somehow. I didn't know how to pick myself up again. All I could see were more and more problems and unbearable pain. I got stuck on what had happened and how my life had been pulled out from under me. I still feel that way.

"It was tough on my family too. I kept pushing them away each time they tried to help. I felt that they would be better off without me.

"I felt so useless. I couldn't get anything done. Even simple things seemed impossible. The depression has lessened since I started on this new medication. But there is still no way I can control pain like I did in the surgery. Sometimes, I'm even afraid of pain and afraid of doing anything that might make it worse. I don't want to get knocked down again."

At that moment, I looked over at Sarah. She still looked like she wanted to fight. "You did it once, Suzanne. You must know that you could do it again, if you want to." Now, Sarah was sounding just like the insurance adjuster she hated so much.

"I want to get that strength back too, Sarah," I said, not wanting to take her bait. "That is why I'm here, with all of you. But if you think that I can just snap my fingers and be able to do what I did before, you're wrong. I can't even imagine being able to control pain like I did before. And you couldn't do it either. Let's face it. You're all in here for a reason too."

Mike stepped in. "Well, well, let's not get so worked up there, superwoman. I am not sure that I like the sound of that. Maybe we can do more than you think."

Ashley smiled. "Let's put her to the test. Maybe she can't do it herself right now, but she sure can talk. Let her show us what she knows and we'll be the judge."

Mike let out a wide grin. "I like the sound of that. We sure need something to get us going here."

With Mike egging us on, the stage was set. The challenge was on.

CHAPTER FIVE

Our Fighting Spirits

Now, we were all in a better mood. Story after story followed. We enjoyed getting to know each other a little better. It felt good knowing we were all in this together.

We talked past Saturday night and well into Sunday morning. After returning to my room, I lay there on my hospital bed for hours. I was exhausted, yet my mind was still racing. My emotions started to churn. Images haunted me – the fall outside my office; the trip to the hospital; disappointments as each specialist told me there was no cure; visiting a lawyer to sell my practice. I had been through hell since my fall and was reliving the chain of events that had brought me to this place. My head pounded. Tears drenched my pillow. Sleep finally took over.

Fortunately, some of my strength and clarity returned over the next few days. This helped me decide to teach my new friends some of what I knew. I wanted to help them. I knew the support from Ashley, Sarah, and Mike would also help me. We had become close in our short time together. If I could help build them up, their renewed strength couldn't help but rub off on me. That is one of the common benefits of inpatient pain programs, I have come to learn.

It was late Thursday afternoon when we gathered again in Mike's room. My friends wanted to jump right in and learn how to become masters over their pain. "Show me the way," said Sarah. "This pain has had its last day pushing me around."

Sarah was in for some surprises, though. My first lesson proved a little disheartening for her. "Sarah, I like your fighting spirit, but let's not start off on the wrong foot. Fighting won't work here. Believe it or not, fighting pain actually makes it worse, not better."

I let this sink in a little, then went on. "When you go to war with pain, pain always wins. The harder you fight, the stronger it gets. It's as though it can use your own anger and willpower against you. This idea surprised me, back when I was preparing for surgery. I wanted to overpower the pain, just as you do. Yet, each time I tried to dominate my pain, it quickly rose up to defeat me."

"I'm lost," said Ashley. I could tell from their blank expressions that Mike and Sarah were also bewildered.

"It was confusing for me too, at first. If you think about it, though, it does make sense. Remember last Saturday night? We talked about how stress can make pain stronger. Well, this is true for stresses that hit us, like losing a job, fighting with our husbands, or reliving memories from our accidents. It is also true for the stresses we create ourselves, like getting angry and wanting to fight back.

"Stress is a physical thing. Our hearts pump faster, our breathing becomes quicker, muscles tense up, including our injured ones, and our bodies get ready for action. These things kick in automatically as soon as our brains and bodies react to strong emotions.

"These stress reactions are not usually a problem for the uninjured parts of our bodies. Our healthy muscles can tense up without becoming painful. Look at the stress we put our hearts under when we exercise. But, what do you think happens to our damaged necks and backs? When those injured areas become tense, our pain flares up. It's like throwing gas on a fire.

"For me, my neck and head are more sensitive to pain flare-ups than my injured back. When my neck pain increases, wicked headaches are soon to follow. So if I tense up, for whatever reason, I get more pain in my neck and head, not less."

"So you are saying that fighting creates stress," said Mike, "and that stress leads to tension and more pain. I guess that makes sense."

"This still doesn't seem right," protested Sarah. "I get mad so easily, and I want to fight back. My pain kills me sometimes."

"It does for me, too, Sarah. And I feel like fighting back. I'm sure we all do. But pain is not the enemy really. My injured body is not against me. It doesn't want to suffer. My body is hurt. It needs to be cared for and strengthened, not hurt more."

I paused to look at Mike and Ashley, and then at Sarah. Empty stares were all around me. They were still confused. So I tried to explain a little more.

"When our pain flares up, we feel like we are under attack – like it is picking a fight with us. It creates an instant urge in us to strike back. We want to defend ourselves against this attack. Our bodies get ready for this fight with tension and adrenaline. And this is the dangerous part. It is this tension and adrenaline that triggers more pain – the opposite of what we want."

Ashley looked up from her notes. "But our bodies *are* hurting us."

"Not really, Ashley. I don't think our bodies are attacking us, even though it feels this way. The pain is there as our bodies try to protect and heal us, the best way they can. There is no intent to harm. Fighting may feel like the only way to react. But, how could we possibly win a war against ourselves?"

Mike was smirking. We all stared at him wondering what he could be thinking during such a serious discussion. "This almost sounds funny," he said. "Like George from Seinfeld. Each time he tried to make things better, he ended up making them worse."

Our comic relief did not last long, however. Sarah was close to tears. "This is not funny. It's hopeless. You say we can't fight. Are we just supposed to just give up and die?"

"*Sarah* – Sarah," I replied. "Let me explain. Please.

"You are right; fighting does seem like the only way. No one would argue with that. The problem is that it doesn't work; at least it didn't for me. I needed another way. Now don't laugh, but learning how to relax, physically and mentally is what worked for me. Relaxation is the opposite of stress, even the stress caused by pain. In fact, if I can get relaxed, I don't even feel like fighting."

Sarah seemed a little calmer. I was trying my best to be reassuring and patient with her. It was taking a lot out of me, though. But I pushed on.

"My first technique was an old one called progressive relaxation. It has been around for ages. I told you about this in my story. Progressive relaxation involves going through each part of your body, first tensing, then releasing and letting each muscle become totally limp. As you work through your body, each part becomes relaxed and you can feel a wave of gentle warmth wash over you. I think we will be learning this soon in our program.

"This method was not designed to control pain, though; at least not in the usual sense. In fact, this technique is not really about pain. I used it to focus on me and my body. I wanted to create a new way of feeling – calm, relaxed, and almost sleepy – the opposite of a fighting mood. The amazing thing was that when my tension went away, my neck slowly became less aggravated and it didn't hurt as much. And I felt I had a little control."

Then I stopped talking for a moment. I could see that their eyes were starting to glaze over – again. "Ashley, are you there?" I asked.

"Yeah, I'm here. I know what you're saying but I don't really like it. I've tried these relaxation exercises. My doctors and therapists are always telling me to relax and slow down. This doesn't come easy when I'm really hurting. I need to move, to do something, to catch up on all the things that don't get done. I'm behind on everything."

"When my pain gets really bad," added Sarah, "it makes me mad. Just like what you're saying. Resting, relaxing, they just make me notice my pain more. And then I get even more worked up. How useful is that?"

"Both of you are right on the mark," I said. "And I think you're seeing just how hard it is to gain some control over pain. Remember though, relaxation is just the starting point. There's more.

"The night before surgery, I followed the progressive relaxation with an imagery technique. This can produce a deep rest for your injured body; it's almost a cleansing of all the tension. In my mind, I imagined all the detailed steps to the surgery. I could see it happening and imagined that it would all work out, and work out perfectly. I also wanted to boost my confidence, since I was a bit nervous about the next day's surgery.

"This type of mental practice is used by athletes as they work on their form and prepare for each competition. Golfers, for example, picture a perfect swing. They imagine in precise detail how each arm and leg is positioned, how each movement feels, and how each shot will go exactly as planned. Golfers don't focus on removing bad habits, they zero in on the technique they want to perfect. Adding a positive usually works much better than trying to remove a negative. And there is less resistance."

"Yeah, but what do we actually do?" asked Mike.

"Can't we just go at it directly and use these methods to take the pain away? This would be so much easier."

"It sure would be, Ashley, but I don't think it works that way. If you think about it, it is hard to imagine the absence of pain, or even the absence of anything. But, you can imagine the presence of certain feelings or sensations. For example, it would be almost impossible to imagine walking without a limp. What would that even feel like? But, you could picture and feel your legs moving in a perfect flow.

"For me, I needed to become totally absorbed in these images and feelings. I think it is this immersion that creates the deep calm. When I focused on the memories of my daughter's birthday party, I was almost able to relive them, in slow motion. I could remember my daughter's face, filled with joy and laughter. I could feel my face get flushed as I soaked up her excitement.

"Sorry," I laughed. "I am getting carried away. Pretty soon you're going to be calling me Drama Queen."

"Keep going," said Mike. "But don't get too deep on us." Sarah nodded in agreement.

"Okay…the pain sensations did break through from time to time, of course. I became aware of them and paid close attention to what they were like – the sharpness, the pulling, pushing, and stretching of parts inside my stomach. I knew what Dr. Grace was doing, so these sensations didn't scare me. I tried to be like an observer watching what was happening inside of me and around the room. Then I would drift back to the memories of my daughter's party.

"If a sharp pain breaks through, you don't want to panic or try to force it away. You want to let it come, check it out, decide if you need to do anything about it, then let it go. This requires a clear, strong mind, as you can imagine. I had it then…I wish I had it now." My throat tightened. Tears were on the verge of breaking through. I was starting to lose it.

I tried to compose myself and carry on, hoping my voice didn't break, hoping my moist eyes were not too obvious to everyone.

"It doesn't work to go head to head against our pain. We should try to reduce pain by removing as many of the aggravations as we can. We have all talked about how fighting can make our pain worse. Lack of sleep is another big aggravator. Without proper sleep, our injured bodies are not able to recover from even one day's pain. We don't want pain from the next day to pile on top. Pain can easily grow out of control that way.

"Stress is another big aggravator. Stress can weaken us and irritate our injured bodies. Short-term stress is not a real danger. But stress that goes on, day after day – like financial problems when you can't work, or battles with insurance companies – can knock us down and keep us there."

Sarah got up and started to pace. She was really fuming this time. "I know you are right. But, whenever I hear about stress and pain in the same sentence, it makes my blood boil."

Sarah was in the middle of a long war with her car insurance company and had been under attack for the previous two and a half years. She had had a hard life with the death of her son ten years ago, the loss of her nursing career after her accident, and the breakup of her marriage last year. Since that time, she had been struggling to cope with pain, losses, and the care of her three young daughters. The insurance doctors had an easy time, though, denying the reality of her injuries. One psychiatrist wrote that her chronic pain was caused by a delayed grief reaction from the death of her son. An orthopedic surgeon, also hired by her insurance adjuster, said that her complaints were probably due to family stress, not any physical cause.

Fortunately, Sarah's physical medicine specialist and psychologist stood up for her. They pointed out she had shown no evidence of pain, disability, or unusual family stress in the two years prior to her car accident. Sarah had a solid record of achievement in college. Her work record at the hospital was flawless. She had only taken two weeks of bereavement time from work after her son's death. Her doctors wrote that her chronic pain symptoms matched perfectly with the symptom patterns of millions of other patients in pain and were able to provide scientific references to back up their opinions. Sarah's insurance adjuster had to back down and reinstate her benefits. Sarah won this battle. But she still felt overwhelmed and always on edge. She never knew when her adjuster would strike again.

"I know this is a very touchy subject for you, Sarah," I said. "For the past fifty years, people have been denying the existence of chronic pain. A favorite tactic has been to blame the injured person and blame any type of stress in her life. Before the MRI was invented, some doctors used to think that multiple sclerosis was caused either by stress or by an individual's weak personality. Now, the evidence from MRI studies is very clear. Stress can aggravate symptoms, of course, just as it can for any type of illness. But, stress is not the cause."

"I understand what you are saying," said Sarah, settling a little. "But it still makes me upset. I am sure that the stress from my marriage problems made it harder for me to cope with my pain. And it probably triggered many pain flare-ups. But, the insurance adjuster and lawyers are still trying to use it to cut me off."

"But, Sarah," followed Mike, "didn't your marriage breakdown come after your accident?"

"That's right," said Ashley. "If it wasn't for your car accident, I bet you and your husband would still be together."

"Maybe so," said Sarah. "Who knows?"

"If you think about it," I said, "the loss of your marriage actually adds to your credibility. To me, it makes perfect sense. Of course, serious injuries, long-term pain, limitations, and depression would interfere with anybody's marriage. How could it not? This is especially true when it is the wife that is injured. Husbands, I think, have a much harder time coping with all the extra duties they have to take over. When children are involved, it is often too much for them."

Mike added, "If I was on a jury, it would make sense to me, too. Even if your marriage was shaky before your accident, and I am not saying it was, stress from a long-lasting injury could be the last straw."

Mike paused, then added. "Sarah, if you try to cover up these stresses, the insurance company will find a way to use that against you as well. My buddies in the union don't think too highly of lawyers and insurance companies. They say that they will keep throwing shit against the wall until something sticks."

"It's true, Sarah," I said. "It will only hurt you if you try and hide the truth. There *are* some stresses in your life that can make your pain worse. That's true for all of us."

"Since our injuries started," said Mike, "our lives have been full of stresses – being out of work, financial troubles, stress in our families, endless appointments and treatments – you name it. And that's not even counting the battles with lawyers and insurance companies. I have workers' compensation on my back."

"All this negativity is so depressing," said Ashley. "I thought we were talking about positive things, like controlling pain. I want to be able to control pain like Suzanne did with her surgery. I know my life is out of control, but does my pain have to be out of control, too?"

That comment stopped my heart for a second. Ashley just put her finger on something very important, not only for me, but for each of us. I was trying to sort out why I could not control my pain the way I did during the operation. But, I was going around in circles and not getting to the heart of it. Soon, with the help of Ashley's insight, this would all make perfect sense to me.

• • •

Over the next few weeks, Ashley, Sarah, and Mike practiced what I taught them. They were curious about these strange techniques. And for the most part, their curiosities allowed them to sidestep their urges to fight back.

Success came easy for them, in the early stages. They learned to enjoy the relaxation exercises that I had shown them and the ones they learned in the program. From their experiences with relaxation, they were able to understand its power. Relaxation helped to reduce the tension that kept aggravating their pain symptoms. It soothed them when they got upset and helped to lessen their irritability and fatigue. They found that their pain symptoms didn't get to them as much. Surprisingly, they felt a little tougher and more resilient. Who would have thought that you could get stronger by fighting less? Maybe Gandhi was right after all.

The imagination exercises allowed them to apply the relaxation experience to a variety of problems. Each imaginary journey could be tailored to a specific goal, like the golfer striving for the perfect swing, or the basketball player, the perfect free throw. Ashley liked to imagine a journey from memory. She would picture the walks on the beach she used to enjoy with her husband near their family cottage. This helped her to unwind during the day when her pain levels would build. She used this technique to avoid some of the flare-ups that would send her to bed rest for days at a time. The peace she felt with these memories spilled over and helped lessen some of her irritable bowel symptoms. (Irritable bowel symptoms are common in people with chronic pain caused by fibromyalgia.)

Mike would imagine himself going out on the perfect date. He had lost self-confidence after his injuries and had convinced himself that no woman would be interested in someone who was disabled and not working. These anxious ruminations would eat away at him, wear him down, and trigger repeated flare-ups of pain. On these imaginary journeys, he imagined himself on wild and fun-filled dates. He practiced how he would ask each woman out on a date, how he would tell her about himself, and how she might respond. He was able to fine-tune the best approach for him and feel some hope for getting back into dating again.

He became more outgoing and more confident. This was a surprise for us, since he was already a friendly and social guy. We didn't know he was so anxious inside. With relaxation and these practice dates, he started to experience fewer anxiety attacks, fewer physical setbacks, and began to feel less like the "cripple" he used to call himself.

The benefits did not come as easily for Sarah. She had understood the concept of not trying to overpower her pain. In practice, however, her own needs and feelings got the best of her. She had learned the basics of relaxation and enjoyed the peaceful feelings in her mind and body. She had different ideas, though, about how to make these benefits work for her.

She thought if she could relax and settle her pain down, then she would be free of physical limitations and free to be active, like she had been prior to her injuries.

This was especially problematic when she would go home on weekend passes from the pain program. There, she would go through the relaxation and imagery exercises, feel better, then try and vacuum her whole house. This didn't work, of course. At other times, she thought that she would catch up with a day of gardening. Predictably, her pain symptoms returned with a fury.

I tried to explain to her that overexertion undid the benefits of the relaxation. By forcing her body to vacuum or garden, she was once again at war with her body. Whatever tension she released with the relaxation exercise was quickly brought back by her forceful efforts. Sarah did not want to hear this, though. She had always been a physical person. She coped with the stresses in her life by distracting herself and boosting her battered self-esteem through productive physical activity. This worked for her after her son died and until she was injured. Afterward, when pain and stress built up, she still tried to work it off physically. This only triggered more pain and more stress. Unfortunately, each struggle made the noose tighter and tighter.

Like many people, Sarah could not accept chronic pain in her life. She suffered from too many losses already. Nor could she accept the physical limitations created by her pain and injuries. She continued to fight against them, even when it was clear that the fighting only caused more pain. The flare-ups of pain would knock her down. When they subsided even a little, she would launch into more activity. Unfortunately, it would take another year and a bout of serious depression before she could even begin to face the truth.

CHAPTER SIX

Emerging from the Fog

The fog thinned for me, after listening to Ashley talk about control. The other night, she had asked why she couldn't control her pain, even with her life out of control. To her, control over her life was, and should be, separate from her capacity to control pain. She wanted to learn how to control her pain first, then work on getting her life back. This made perfect sense. The ongoing pain and limitations were the reasons for her life going out of control, so she wanted to eliminate the obstacles and return to a normal life. This is how most people think about pain, injury, or any kind of illness. Cure the cause, then you are free to move on.

My mind kept racing over the next few weeks in the pain program. I made many trips to the pain psychologist's office to share my ideas with him. Gradually, I began to see that this process of control might work differently than I had thought. If your life is out of control, you are living in a high-stress situation. This means that your pain and injuries are always being aggravated. How can they settle down under these circumstances? You can try to reduce the stress and tension by relaxing and slowing down. But, as soon as you open your eyes and start thinking again, the stresses are back in your life, and in full force. The next time you open the mail or get another call from the collection agency, you are reminded of being out of work. Letters from the bank tell you that your debt is mounting. The stress is around every corner, and everywhere you turn.

I started to see I had to regain control over my life first. Then I might have a chance at controlling my pain. Before I had the surgery done, my life was going just as I had planned. I was working, in good health, full of energy, independent, and able to concentrate on my techniques. The pain control techniques did not do the job by themselves, though. They needed an operator with a strong, determined, and clear mind. That was me at that time. I did not have a lot of stress, uncertainty, or loss in my life; my daily life stresses weren't very intense and generally under control.

Since the fall outside my dental office, my life had controlled me. When I lost my disability benefits and then my dental practice, whatever control I did have was gone. These losses sent my pain soaring. I was raging inside, but I felt unable to do anything about it. The insurance company had all the power. I felt like an insect, squashed without hesitation. Did they even consider what their actions would do to me? They must have known that by cutting me off, I would not be able to pay my bills and would lose my practice. Did they think that this stress would strengthen me? It didn't; it crushed me and sent me into a deep despair. Now I was disabled, not only from my physical injuries, but also from depression. There was no way I could return to work then. How could I?

This whole pattern appeared much clearer to me after telling the story to my new friends. When it was first happening, though, I didn't make any connection between the stress caused by my insurance company and my worsened injuries. All I could feel was the increase in my pain. I was angry, yes, but it was my severe neck pain and headaches that floored me. I didn't know why it was so severe and I didn't really care why. I just wanted some fast relief. My family doctor helped by increasing my pain medication.

I continued to deteriorate, though. My sleep worsened. I became so irritable that my family was ready to disown me. I did not get much for the sale of my dental practice because I was so desperate to sell. And when it was gone, I thought my career in dentistry was over. Who am I? I am not a dentist anymore. I don't have an income; I can't even support myself. I lost all hope; nothing seemed possible anymore. My pain got worse, with one flare-up merging into the next. All I cared about was some kind of relief.

My doctor tried to tell me I was depressed, but I got defensive with her. I didn't want to hear about depression and stress, I only wanted her to find a cure for this endless torture. She tried to explain that depression was making my pain worse, but I didn't understand her thinking. I didn't even listen to her, really. Now, I know what she was talking about. She was trying to explain the chain reaction that had started with my injury. The injury led to prolonged pain, loss of work, loss of benefits, insomnia, and depression, which led to more pain. My doctor knew I could not straighten out this whole mess by focusing only on pain relief. Taking more and more pain medication would only result in an additional problem: that of addiction.

As the fog lifted, I could see the stresses that were making my pain escalate. To obtain any kind of lasting relief for my pain, I had to find a way to climb out of this hole and reduce all these aggravations. If it were possible to cure my pain and return to work, this clearly would have been an easier route for me. Such cures have yet to be discovered, however.

Throughout the rest of the pain program, I kept testing these ideas with fellow patients and staff. They all agreed that it boiled down to me regaining some kind of control over my life. That was the common thread. My husband was trying to tell me that for some time. He hated seeing me in such a helpless state. He was the laid-back one; I was the one who always had the ideas and the drive.

My husband would joke that I was the control freak in the family. After I lost my practice though, he said that I had just given up. I blasted him for those comments and accused him of not understanding the severity of my pain. It took me a while to see what was really happening. My pain was severe; I knew deep inside he understood, and better than anyone. Whenever I didn't want to face things, I would accuse whoever would listen of not knowing what it was really like for me. That was my defense; I was quick to use it with anyone who dared to challenge me.

It took until the end of the pain program before I was able to see the whole picture. I knew, then, what I had to do. First, I had to find solid footing so that I could stop falling. I needed a secure financial base. Since I could no longer work – now for a combination of reasons – I decided to go after my insurance company and make them own up to their responsibilities. I had a talk with my lawyer, but he was of no help. As I suspected, he was only interested in my lawsuit against the owner of the building where I had fallen and became injured. His plan was to wait until the time was right (whenever that would have been), negotiate a settlement, and collect his fee. How I survived until then was my problem, not his.

I ditched this lawyer and looked for one who would help me with my disability insurer and help me with my lawsuit. Both of these problems needed expert legal help. After a few interviews with lawyers, I settled on one whom was willing to spend some time with me and who was able to explain the strengths and weaknesses of my case in a language I could understand. He agreed to go after my disability insurer first and have my monthly benefits restored.

My case was a good one, as I understood it. The medical evidence was strong. My family doctor, medical specialists, and psychologist had outlined my diagnoses and had stated that I was unable to go back to dentistry. The insurance doctors and adjuster were not convinced, however. They kept writing in their reports that there was not enough evidence to honor my claim.

At first, I didn't understand what the adjuster and insurance doctors were up to. The evidence was there, why wouldn't they accept it? This was driving me crazy.

I felt like they were holding all the cards. The insurance company was a billion dollar corporation. What power did I have?

The missing link, my lawyer explained, was a detailed description of how my injuries actually limited my ability to work. My doctors had diagnosed my neck, back, and head injuries, my chronic pain, and my depression. What they had not explained, though, was the connections between my diagnoses, my inability to work as a dentist, and how my health would worsen if I tried to return to dentistry. It had to be clearly documented that if I tried doing dental work my pain levels and depression would worsen, causing me further harm.

My lawyer overcame these weaknesses by writing letters to each of my doctors. He asked them to answer specific questions in his letters. Then, he organized the information from the previous reports and my doctors' answers to his questions. He was then able to explain all the reasons for my inability to work. Each of my limitations were spelled out and connected to my fall and to the injuries. He made sure that both my physical and psychological injuries were fully explained.

I was worried that the insurance company would think depression was my only problem and that I could really work if I had wanted to. My lawyer explained that my physical injuries, my chronic pain, and my depression were all serious conditions and legitimate reasons for a person to be unable to work. In terms of the law, the dark ages were coming to a close. Companies could no longer blame people when they suffered from depression. In fact, depression and anxiety are very common reactions to any type of chronic illness and represent added reasons why individuals cannot work.

Within a few months, the insurance company relented. They started paying me regular benefits in full. This was not enough to live on, of course. My benefits were much lower than my income as a dentist had been, but it was a start. I could pay off some of my debts. More importantly, I didn't feel like I was sinking any more. I was at least able to tread water and to start looking around for shore.

It took a few more months for my lessened stress to pay off physically. My husband actually noticed before I did. I became less irritable, had fewer pain flare-ups, and I seemed a little brighter each day. I even started to think of new possibilities. Predictably, he started in with the jokes again.

I became able to think more clearly as I emerged from the fog of pain, medication, and despair. And with the help of my rehab psychologist, I was able to boil down my problems to the two big ones: physical pain and the loss of my career. I now had a little financial safety, which lessened some of my stress. I had confidence and trust in my new lawyer. This also helped me to feel some control in my life. With these stresses reduced, and the careful usage of my new longer-acting pain medications, my pain levels felt more manageable. A return to full-time dentistry was still out of the question, though; this meant that my second biggest problem was still standing before me.

I soon found out that a resolution to this problem would require much sorting out. The practical steps were the easy ones. I pestered my doctors with endless questions. What were my restrictions? When will they go away? (I don't think I will ever stop asking this one.) What would happen if I just pushed myself, took more medication, and tried to return to work no matter how I felt? This was Sarah's favorite approach, which unfortunately caused her much agony.

Some of the answers to these questions I already knew. I kept asking them, though; hoping somehow that the next time I asked the answer would be different. I was always hoping for a cure, the miracle that would return me to my former life. My doctors were straight with me about my limitations and my future. I appreciated their honesty, but their doses of reality were hard to stomach. In fact, throughout this whole process my emotions were churned, over and over. Old and powerful feelings of grief were stirred up and exposed. This was one of the hardest parts.

Gradually, a consensus emerged among my doctors. I told them I did not want to give up dentistry all together. They told me I might be able to do some part-time teaching or even hands-on dental work, but only for very short periods of time. This would mean more pain flare-ups, of course, and regular periods of inactivity in between. It would be necessary, they said, to avoid an accumulation of pain, which occurs when flare-ups occur back to back, with no time to recover between bouts. This is the pattern, which leads to higher and higher pain levels, insomnia, depression, and a life out of control. This was the really harmful part. I had been there and did not want to go back.

To test my limits, I arranged to do some volunteer work in the student clinic at the dentistry school. I started doing three afternoons per week, three hours each time. My duties were mainly supervisory, although I did have to demonstrate certain procedures from time to time. I experienced more flare-ups and occasionally I missed whole weeks when bad ones set in. When my seventy year-old mother had to go in for surgery, for example, my stress level increased temporarily and more flare-ups were triggered. The dental school could not complain too much, though. They were getting my help for free.

Over the next four to five months, my strength and stamina increased. I was able to manage the routine of three afternoons per week with little time missed. Then, I caught a lucky break and was offered a paid position as a part-time instructor. This was a big boost for me. For the first time in ages, I felt like I was worth something. A little independence felt really good.

This employment didn't help my finances, though. I soon found out that any money I earned had to be returned to my disability insurer, at least until I surpassed sixty percent of my former income, which may have been never. My heart sank; the dense fog reappeared. I spent the next weekend in bed, defeated, again. It all felt so wrong.

I was angry and hurt. The old feelings of powerlessness crept back into my life. It was different this time, though. I had some energy reserves built up from my recent successes. I was able to step back and see what was happening to me. The flare-ups were painful, as always, but I knew what had triggered them and what had knocked me down. I also knew, now more than ever, that I had to get the insurance system out of my life.

CHAPTER SEVEN

One Year Later

One year later and we were all back at the hospital for a follow-up assessment. It was not quite as dismal as I remembered. The green paint and the odor of disinfectant were just as intense. There was a familiar warmth, though.

As the elevator opened onto the second floor, I spotted Mike right away. He gave me a real bear hug and couldn't wait to tell me how he had been doing.

It had been a difficult year for Mike, at least initially. His life was going nowhere. He felt like he was treading water for too long. Anxiety about his future made him angry and defensive in his dealings with the workers' compensation board. This was unlike him. Yet, more conflict and tension had built up, triggering repeated pain flare-ups. He felt that the board had all the power. What Mike did not realize, though, was that his caseworker had also felt helpless, not knowing how to help him.

Fortunately, Mike got the opportunity to work with a rehab psychologist, Dr. Turner, following a referral from the pain program. Mike was not crazy, nor were there any psychological causes for his pain. But he did need help to sort out a new direction for himself. He also needed help to understand the workers' compensation system and how he could best work within it. Being angry and defensive had not been helpful to anyone. It had led to a stalemate, with no end in sight. Just more treading water, more stress, and more pain.

Mike and Dr. Turner started by reviewing reports from each of Mike's doctors. They were looking for clear opinions about his injured shoulder and about Mike returning to his former job in construction. Some of his doctors had not been clear on this latter point, so Mike scheduled further visits with them. Gradually, all the reports came together in agreement that Mike could no longer work in his chosen field. This was hard for him to accept. He had not known any other type of work. Construction had been a hard job, but it was familiar, it paid reasonably well, and he was good at it. Without construction to go back to, his future seemed uncertain and threatening.

Mike was almost out of breath as he recounted these details. I knew his story was just warming up, though. He was frightened at having to confront the loss of his familiar job in construction. But, Dr. Turner helped him to see that a better work future could be possible for him, if only he would cooperate with his caseworker. The caseworker was looking for some direction from Mike and was open to any ideas that would resolve the conflict between them.

As Mike learned more about the compensation system, he discovered there was funding available for him to be retrained and to find a new line of work. Most importantly, his loss of earnings benefits would continue while he went through this vocational rehabilitation.

This was a bright ray of hope for him. He started soon thereafter, with some academic upgrading courses, including two grade twelve courses that would give him a high school diploma. School was difficult at first. Long days of taking notes led to many flare-ups of his shoulder pain. The stresses at school were also overwhelming, since he had little confidence that he could do well in school.

He had been doing better by the time we met. Each success at school helped to boost his confidence and his energy. Pain flare-ups were less frequent and not as severe. He started to feel that a decent future might be possible for him. His plan was to finish the high school courses, then enroll in a construction technology and business program that would train him for work in building supply stores. These new possibilities excited him. The work duties would be compatible with his chronic shoulder pain and any wage loss would be made up by workers' compensation.

Mike started to ask me how I was doing, when Ashley squeezed in between us. Both Mike and I laughed and then smiled. Ashley looked great. She seemed naturally happy, energetic, and very glad to see us.

I was pleasantly surprised. Ashley lost that forced-smile look. I was glad to see her looking so well, but was confused at the same time. I heard that she endured some serious setbacks over the past year. I knew her health had worsened. The pain and fatigue from her neck injury and fibromyalgia had become more debilitating. Yet, here she was looking better than I had ever seen her.

Ashley explained it was a roller coaster year for her. Yes, she did have more pain, but that had lessened over the past few months. She had become pregnant. Pregnancy, at least so far, had actually helped her pain. She knew she had to be careful and take better care of herself. She had stopped pushing so hard. Those around her were always offering to help do things for her. Even her husband was now doing the laundry and helping with meals. She was able to rest more, which helped restore some of her energy. Her flare-ups had lessened, even the overwhelming ones caused by her fibromyalgia.

She was thrilled to be pregnant. Ashley and her husband had been putting off starting a family since becoming injured in the car accident. They had been waiting for her to feel better, but that had not been happening. When she started to get worse, they were forced into a tough decision. They talked it over with her family doctor and specialists. It became clear that it was now or never, so they decided to start a family right away.

The doctors had told Ashley that her chances of being able to work again were slim. They could not guarantee that she would be able to care for a child, either. Yet, Ashley knew that she had to try. The thought of going through life without having children was unthinkable. She knew it was the right decision. Since she had become pregnant, she felt even more certain.

As we listened to Ashley, I noticed Mike could not hold back the toothy grin on his face. "Mike, you sure look happy to hear Ashley's news," I said.

"I am. Ashley is pregnant and looks great. But, I have been waiting to tell you all some extra good news of my own. I met a new friend in school, over the past month, and we have started dating. Her name is Karen and I really like her. I know it is still early, but maybe a family is in the cards for us down the road."

"I didn't know that pregnancy was contagious," I said. Before I could finish my sentence, Ashley turned toward the other side of the room and shouted for Sarah to come over and join us.

Sarah came right over. She noticed us all smiling and asked what was up. We filled her in on the pregnancy and budding romance, teasing Mike in the process.

"I wish that I could join the fun. It has been pretty tough for me this year; actually it's been difficult for many years now. But you probably don't want to hear all about my doom and gloom. Actually, it is not all gloom."

"Of course, we do, Sarah," said Ashley. "Tell us everything. We are all in this together, you know." We then moved over to a quiet table in the corner.

Sarah had not been the same person since being hit by the drunk driver. Chronic pain had changed her, as it had changed each of us. Sarah did not like the person she had become: sad, quick to anger, and in many ways still trying to fight her way out. She suffered from repeated flare-ups. It was difficult to slow down with a busy household and young children to manage. Increases in pain stirred up waves of despair regarding her lost career and looming divorce. Sarah became exhausted and sunk into a deep depression. Next came an overdose of pills. She was rushed to hospital and admitted to the mental health wing.

"This was my lowest point," explained Sarah. "Everyone would know I'm crazy, I thought. The insurance company would have all the evidence they needed to prove that my pain was all in my head. I figured I was really done this time.

"But the hospital turned out to be a blessing in disguise. A social worker came to see me shortly after my admission. Evelyn had previously worked in a pain program and figured me out right away. She knew I wasn't crazy. She knew my chronic pain was real. She knew I was still angry about my pain and about the drunk driver that had ruined my life. Surprisingly, Evelyn told me I also felt powerless and weak. My angry front hadn't fooled her. Then she shocked me by asking me what I was going to do about it.

"At first, I didn't know what she meant. She knew I had injuries and pain that could not be cured. She readily admitted that. She knew I had been fighting hard to recover. But then she asked what I was going to do about my ruined life. I was more confused than ever. So, as usual I got all defensive with her. I told her there was nothing I could do. Then I accused her of not understanding how hard it was for me."

"Hey, I do that too," I interrupted. We all smiled.

"But before I really got going with this, Evelyn cut me off. 'This is not going anywhere right now. I will prepare my initial report. You will be able to see in black and white that I do know what you have been going through. I will give you a copy of my report and will send copies to your lawyer and insurance company. Then if you still don't trust me, our work will be over.'"

"Wow," said Ashley. "She's a tough one. What did you do?"

"Well, I read her report and it seemed that she was being straight with me. Then I sort of gave in and started listening to her. We came back to her original question: 'What are you going to do to stop feeling so angry and weak?'

"Evelyn explained that my feelings were so strong that they were triggering flare-up after flare-up, wearing me down, and making me feel even more helpless. My answers were not working, according to Evelyn. Her answer was that I had to come up with some non-physical ways of feeling strong and useful. I had to find some way of moving forward in my life."

"This sounds kind of familiar, Sarah. Hadn't you heard that advice before?" Mike was goading her, gently.

"Yes, Mike, I had." Sarah let out a slow smile. "But, shut up for a moment and let me talk.

"So I joined a group in town that was trying to change the laws against drunk driving. This was a cause that I believed in. My anger was useful there, and I started feeling like I could accomplish something again. Evelyn liked this idea. And as I got a little stronger and less depressed, I started feeling more ambitious.

"In our counseling sessions, we would talk a lot about how my insurance company had been treating me. I explained that my benefits and many of the treatments and medications that could have helped me had been denied. She knew that I was also concerned about the many other car accident victims who had been treated the same way by their insurers. Her response was the same. 'What are you going to do about it? Stewing in your own anger and flaring up your pain are not helping."

"I can't believe this Evelyn," I said. "She's relentless."

"But wait, I haven't told you the best part yet. I gradually got more confident – and bolder – the more I talked to Evelyn. I met some interesting people. You wouldn't believe how many people have been hurt by drunk drivers, and how many people have been screwed by their insurance companies. So a few of us started meeting together to talk. At first, all we would do was complain. Then I started acting like Evelyn. I confronted our group with the challenge to stop complaining and to do something. I became the ringleader; can you believe it?

"Our group decided to do something radical, to change some things. Many people feel that they are alone, trying to fight billion-dollar insurance companies. They feel angry and helpless, just like I felt.

"Our first step was to set up a website, full of true stories about how people in pain have been treated by insurance companies. We did not want to rely on statistics or surveys. We wanted something stronger with real stories and pictures of the people and families that have been hurt. One man in our group has had some professional experience with websites. He helped us a lot.

"My job in this group is to find articles and scientific information about chronic pain that we can put on the website. People need to know chronic pain is never all in your head – it's never just stress. Another part of my job has been to help readers understand what their rights are and how they can defend themselves. I also help people find the right lawyer sometimes. Another woman's job is to promote our site, by discussing it on chat lines, blogs, and through medical and support group email lists."

Sarah took a breath. "I can't believe how well this is all working. I think this can really shake things up and bring some fairness to the people who need it the most. We also help people find pain programs to go to for help – even programs like this one."

All of a sudden, Sarah realized that she was hogging the floor. She became quiet. "I'm sorry, all I've been doing is talking about me."

"That's okay," replied Ashley. "Your stuff sounds really exciting. Maybe I could help out?"

Then, Mike looked straight at me, still smiling. "You know, we haven't heard about you yet."

I couldn't wait to tell them. "I'm happy to say that I, too, had been able to create a bit of a new life for myself. My new lawyer was able to settle my lawsuit and to arrange a buy-out from my long-term disability insurer. The evidence was strong and my doctors showed their willingness to support me if a trial was needed. This helped my lawyer to force a compromise with the insurance lawyers. The insurance and legal system is now out of my life forever. It feels good, believe me.

"My big break, though, happened when I got that volunteer position at the dentistry school. I put myself to the test there. My work was mostly supervisory, but from time to time I was able to demonstrate some procedures to the students. Of course, each time I did anything that took longer than fifteen minutes, I knew that I was in trouble. I would pay a full price later that day. Major flare-ups, believe me. Yet, in the back of my mind, there was this faint hope that if I really pushed, I could work as a dentist again. It took a few months for reality to sink in.

"Luckily for me, there were other options. The director of the dental school liked my work there and offered me a part-time teaching position. It was a good deal. I was still able to work and stay in the dentistry field. I like that. It feels good to get out and be around people again, rather than being stuck at home, depressed.

"I'm not as obsessed anymore, with the loss of my dental practice. I'm not as frightened of being in pain for the rest of my life, either. Of course, that's easier to say now, because my pain is not as severe. I still get flare-ups, just like you guys do. I really can't do much without my pain bringing me down. But my flare-ups happen less often and I can recover faster when they do hit. I feel like I can get on with life a little now, whatever that means."

"So, are you ready to tackle another surgery?" asked Mike, catching me off guard.

"You like to get under my skin, don't you?" I countered, then paused.

"No, I think those days are over. In fact, I can't even imagine being able to do something like that. I know it is possible, at least with that kind of pain – short-term pain, I mean. Pain from surgery is temporary, more like normal pain. It can be overwhelming and severe, but there is a clear end to it. It doesn't grind you down, day after day, month after month, until you have nothing left. We all know chronic pain is a different kind of pain. It's hard to get a handle on, never ending; it's like a slow torture."

I tried to steady my voice. "I'm a different person now. I have been to hell and back. In some ways, though, I am even stronger. I don't mean like before, when I had my surgery done. Back then, I thought I could conquer anything. Now, I look at life a little differently. I understand pain and my body in new ways. I treat them more carefully. They are not separate things, but a part of me, a part of my life."

Ashley broke in, smiling. "That goes double for me. Pregnancy has taught me to take care of my body and to help it to do its work whenever I can."

"Now, now, let's not get all sentimental here," added Sarah, "although, I do agree with you. I still don't like it, but even I am trying to push a little less. Or, as Evelyn would say, push in a useful direction. The work that I am doing with our website has really helped me. My stress has lessened and I get fewer flare-ups. There are at least a few things going right in my life these days."

I saw Mike smile and knew what he was thinking. There were a few things going right in his life too – actually more than a few things. Ashley noticed his smile, then we all lit up a little.

In the background, we heard the program director speak up. It was time to head off. We had to meet with our doctors to have our progress over the past year assessed. "This should be interesting," I thought.

Before we left, Mike stopped us. His voice started to crack as he tried to speak. "Let's try and keep in touch." Then, Mike raised his coffee cup. "A toast to all of us. We sure have come a long way. To next time – to hope – to our new lives."

NOTES

What Is Chronic Pain?

Let's make this very simple.

Chronic pain is basically long-term pain. It can get complicated when parts of your life become disrupted and stressed. But the simplest definition is that pain lasting longer than six months is chronic pain. It can be caused by any type of illness or injury. What makes pain chronic, however, is that it is long-lasting. I will discuss the nature of chronic pain in more detail, but first, I think it is helpful to discuss how it is different from short-term pain.

Short-Term Pain

When you think of pain, you may think about common, everyday experiences. You know that pain hurts, and that some types of pain really hurt. Some are literally unbearable. A bad toothache is a good example. Other pains may be less intense, like a twisted ankle, for instance.

After an injury, the pain sensations usually start to fade. Often, there is something you can do to lessen the intensity. You can rub it, press on it, put on a bandage, or take some medication. Within a short period of time, you can notice changes in your pain. Gradually, you start to feel better. You don't have to endure the pain for very long, and even the knowledge that it is getting better gives you the hope and the strength to persevere. Since it is short-term, the disruption to your life is usually minimal.

The pain of childbirth is a clear example of short-term pain. No one would doubt the severity of the pain involved. Pain from a surgical incision can also be very intense. In both of these instances, there is a known end to the pain. Each day after surgery, the pain gets a little less intense. You know that it is getting better. Soon it will be over.

Short-term pain is called acute pain in medical circles. It can be as severe and debilitating as any other type of pain, but it is not long-lasting. When the pain subsides, you can recover your physical and emotional strength and go about putting your life back in order.

Short-term pain acts like a warning signal; it is a body alarm that tells you that something is wrong. Pain in your chest could be a signal that you are having a heart attack and that you'd better rush to get help. Other examples would include pain from kidney stones or pain from a fractured wrist. The pain is usually followed by a sense of urgency. Your body has been damaged and needs help right away.

A feeling of anxiety usually follows closely behind the pain. The pain may be new and unfamiliar. You may start to worry about the pain. Will it get worse? How bad is the injury? Do you need to get help immediately or can you safely wait and see if it settles down on its own?

Your body will react automatically with anxiety; it is not a reaction that you can plan or choose. Increases in heart rate, blood pressure, breathing, perspiration, and muscle tension are activated. Your body gets ready to take emergency action. Interestingly, you can experience the same pattern of uncontrolled bodily responses even in anticipation of pain. Sitting in a dentist's chair, looking at the large needle that is about to be stuck into your mouth will usually bring about some level of anxiety.

Overall, short-term pain is usually thought of as a good thing; it is a useful warning signal that tells you that something needs your immediate attention. It is a signal that is difficult to ignore. For this reason, it does a good job of getting you energized to take the steps necessary to fix the problem, or get the help you need.

Chronic Pain

Pain is a necessary part of life. Short-term pain, especially, is your body's fire alarm. It is a powerful signal warning you of trouble in your body, forcing you to seek help, to take action.

What would it be like, though, if the fire alarm were stuck on? Imagine how exhausting that would be. As a sufferer of long-term pain, you do not need your imagination here. You know what it is like. You know how often you have gone to doctors and therapists, desperate for someone to shut off your relentless pain. You know the toll that long-term pain has taken on you and your family.

Both long-term pain and short-term pain involve real physical sensations that can vary in intensity. Sometimes these sensations are mild and more of a nuisance to us, and other times they are excruciating. Chronic pain can develop after any type of injury or illness. In some people, repetitive activities in assembly line or computer work can lead to chronic shoulder or wrist pain, as examples. Chronic pain can also develop following a single high-impact trauma, such as a car accident. Neck and back injuries are very common causes of chronic pain. Arthritis is also a common cause.

Another defining feature of chronic pain is its long-term nature. Day after day, month after month, it can gain the power to wear you down, to weaken you, and to disrupt so many parts of your life. On one level, this is very obvious. Of course, long term is long-term. Anyone can see the logic here. Yet, this is not a simple or minor point. When pain becomes chronic, it takes on a whole different character. Its impact on your life can be huge, affecting your ability to enjoy even the simplest moments.

When pain becomes chronic, it means there is no instant cure, no immediate medical fix through surgery or medication. Your life has been changed by your injury or illness. You may suffer from multiple chronic pains caused by multiple injuries. If you were hurt in a car accident, for instance, you may suffer from chronic neck, arm, and back pain, all at the same time. However, with time, treatment, and proper management detailed throughout this book, your pain and suffering can be reduced substantially. Your life will never be the same, though. You can never go back. And, I don't need to tell you this is one of the most challenging parts of any chronic health problem.

Chronic pain is more than just pain. Its long-term nature creates new symptoms, such as poor sleep, fatigue, mood changes, reduced short-term memory, and a variety of new stresses. Drs. Michael Von Korff and Kate Dunn discussed this complexity of chronic pain in a recent review article in the journal *Pain* (2008). To understand how pain affects you, they argued that it is necessary to consider the duration of pain, as well as pain intensity, activity limitations, depressive symptoms and the number of types of pain you experience. Ongoing pain is the cause of these complicated symptoms, which all affect your ability to cope with the pain itself. It becomes a vicious cycle; pain causes stress, which leads to more pain. This is part of what makes chronic pain so complicated and overwhelming for so many people.

The vicious cycle of long-term pain can also lead to major losses and disruptions to you and your family's lives. If chronic pain interferes with your capacity to work, for instance, you may lose your job and have difficulty finding a replacement compatible with your limitations. You may be forced to rely on insurance or government benefits to help you live. As you may know, such benefits can be quite low compared to your work income. The increased stresses, caused by these losses and forced changes to your life, make it all the more difficult to manage your never-ending pain.

When you look at this big picture, you can see that long-term pain is real, physical pain, and much more. This is why chronic pain is often referred to as a syndrome:

chronic pain syndrome (or the more recent term, chronic pain disorder). The word "syndrome" means a collection of symptoms, not just a single one. When pain becomes chronic, it sets off a chain reaction leading to a whole collection of additional symptoms, stresses, losses, limitations, and forced life changes. *Please remember this idea.* It is very important, and we will come back to it again and again with more details and ways to fight back.

Suzanne, Ashley, Sarah, and Mike had to learn, from the chronic pain program and from each other, that their chronic pains were more than just pain. They knew this before they went into the hospital program, but hadn't really put all that information together into a clear understanding of how their injuries and pain had affected their lives. They didn't really connect their pain symptoms with the stresses that were caused by their chronic pain. They were focused only on their pain symptoms and were missing the larger picture. This wider view included all the additional symptoms and stresses that their pain had caused. They came to realize that fighting their pain also meant fighting to get control of the stresses in their life. These two goals had to go hand in hand before they were able to make any real progress toward their recovery. Each of them had to learn how to gain some control over the chronic pain and their disrupted lives.

Suzanne, Ashley, Mike, and Sarah were not alone in their struggle. As they learned in their hospital pain program, chronic pain is a serious worldwide problem.

Chronic Pain Is Recognized Around the World

From research studies over the past fifty years, scientists have learned an enormous amount about the nature of pain and how it affects people. Professors Dennis Turk and Ronald Melzack have put together collections of scientific papers summarizing the latest research on pain. These appear in their books, *Handbook of Pain Assessment* (2001, and an earlier edition from 1992). From these scientific papers, it is known that fifty to seventy percent of people will experience back pain at some point in their lives. Each year, over fifty million North Americans will suffer from pain caused by traumatic injuries, such as car or work accidents. It has also been documented that over forty-five million Americans and Canadians will suffer from muscle pain and over eighty-eight million people will suffer from joint pain. Fortunately, these pain symptoms will be temporary for most of these people.

For many others, though, their pain will not go away with time. In the *Nuprin Pain Report* (one of the first large-scale studies on pain published; Taylor and Curran, 1985) investigators found that over twelve percent of individuals in the United States had experienced pain on at least one hundred and one days of the preceding year. In 1988, research from a Seattle health maintenance organization found that thirty-seven percent of people were suffering from recurrent pain and eight percent reported severe persistent pain (Von Koroff, 1992; Von Koroff, Dworkin, LeReserche and Krugen, 1988). A large-scale investigation from 2001 conducted in fourteen countries found that twenty-two percent of people experienced long-term pain. In this international study, back pain, headaches, and joint pain were found to be the most common types of chronic pain (Gureje, Simon and Von Koroff, 2001). These statistics probably reflect only "the tip of the iceberg," according to world-renowned pain scientists Turk and Melzack (1992), since many people suffer in silence without seeking medical attention.

The scientific literature has clearly documented the high rate and alarming toll caused by chronic pain for people throughout the world. In several studies, long-term pain has been identified as the leading cause of permanent disability and work loss. Dr. John Bonica, considered the "father of pain therapy," estimated that fifty million North Americans experience pain-related disability (Gatchel, 2005; Report of the Commission on Evaluation of Pain, 1986; Vasudevan, 1992). In economic terms, losses of productivity, and the costs of treatment, unemployment, and disability benefits for chronic pain sufferers has been estimated at more than seventy billion dollars per year in the United States alone (Turk and Winter, 2006). This is a driving force for researchers, drug companies, government agencies, and large disability insurers desperate to find a solution to the chronic pain crisis. The United States Congress designated 2001–2010 as the Decade of Pain Control and Research. Pain control has now been recognized as a national and international priority.

Scientists and specialists in this field have recognized chronic pain as a legitimate medical problem for the past fifty years. Yet, it has only been since the early 1990s that chronic pain has been identified as an official diagnostic category: Chronic Pain Disorder (CPD). Since then, disability guidelines have been published by the American Medical Association (AMA). The AMA *Guidelines for the Evaluation of Permanent Impairment* describe chronic pain as a destructive force that can lead to "despair, alienation from family and society, loss of job, isolation, invalidism, and suicidal thoughts. Yet, it is not a psychiatric disorder" (1993, page 15/307).

The AMA guides have also been very clear in stating that chronic pain is not a mental disorder, and not a psychogenic problem. (Psychogenic refers to an injury or illness caused by psychological or emotional factors.) Professors Turk and Melzack go one step further. They review the scientific literature and conclude that the search for a "pain-prone personality" and "psychogenic pain" has been futile. Early psychoanalytic research told us that certain kinds of personality problems could cause pain. This view is now outdated and has been largely abandoned for lack of any scientific evidence. Most pain scientists and doctors in this field now agree that chronic pain is a real and physical health problem that can be aggravated by psychological stress.

There has been significant progress toward the recognition of chronic pain and how, for some people, it can become disabling. Chronic pain has been recognized as a legitimate source of injury and disability by many government disability programs. These include the Social Security Insurance program in the United States and the

Canada Disability Pension program. In fact, claims from individuals who are disabled by chronic pain are higher than claims for many other health problems.

Health, disability, and automobile insurance companies recognize chronic pain. These companies must routinely pay income replacement benefits for individuals with long-term pain when they can no longer work, as well as provide coverage for treatment. This is true for insurance companies and government agencies that provide workers' compensation benefits.

Lawyers have also learned a lot about chronic pain over the years. The evidence in support of the legitimacy of chronic pain is now so overwhelming that it is widely recognized by the courts. Individuals with chronic pain are often unable to work. This creates loss of income and life disruption, which can be compensated by civil lawsuits. Neck and back injuries following car accidents are common causes of chronic pain brought before the courts.

I have discussed in this section how chronic pain is a much more complicated and serious problem than that of short-term pain. Chronic pain is harder to endure; can create secondary health problems such as insomnia, mood changes, and memory interference; and most importantly, it can lead to job loss, financial stress, and marital and family disruption. For some people, almost all aspects of their day-to-day life have been affected. This book is devoted to helping you with your chronic pain *and* with all the related stresses and losses that can be caused by your pain.

• • •

References containing a wealth of additional scientific evidence regarding the nature and extent of chronic pain can be found at the end of this book.

Other scientific articles on almost any health topic
can be found through the PubMed Website:
www.ncbi.nlm.nih.gov/pubmed

What Is Fibromyalgia?

Fibromyalgia is a more complicated form of chronic pain. Just as other illnesses and injuries can develop into long-term pain, so can the illness of fibromyalgia. One of the main symptoms of fibromyalgia is long-term pain. This type of long-term pain can also lead to long-term problems in an individual's life, as can other types of chronic pain. The other main symptoms of fibromyalgia are overwhelming fatigue, sleep dysfunction and cognitive impairment (Sumpton and Moulin, 2008).

Fibromyalgia has been shown to affect two to seven percent of the population of the developed world. And this is just one form of chronic pain. Fibromyalgia is most commonly experienced by women. Symptom onset is usually between the ages of 30 to 55 years of age. Fibromyalgia can also occcur in women and men of younger and older ages, as well as in children. School-age children can experience particularly difficult times with the effects of pain, fatigue and cognitive limitations. School performance, emotional development and relationships with peers can all be affected (Sumpton and Moulin, 2008).

Fibromyalgia is most complicated because the pain symptoms are not just in one part of a person's body. By definition, individuals with fibromyalgia experience widespread body pain. These are real and physical pain sensations that can occur in several parts of the body, all at the same time. The pattern of pain symptoms can vary person to person, but individuals with fibromyalgia will always experience more than one source of pain (Starlanyl, 2009). These sources of pain can appear throughout a person's body. Many patients describe feeling as if a truck has run over them.

Fibromyalgia is also complicated because there can be additional physical symptoms that come with the widespread body pain. With long-term pain, individuals also can experience stiffness, fatigue, numbness and weakness, swelling, cold intolerance, poor sleep, dry eyes, headaches, and bowel problems. The following tables list some of the more common symptoms that can occur in individuals with fibromyalgia. This information was gathered by Dr. Robert Olin from his medical clinic in Sweden. The percentages are based on a survey of over fifteen hundred patients. He presented these findings in a keynote speech at the Seattle Fibromyalgia Conference in 1996. His speech was later summarized in an issue of the *Fibromyalgia Newsletter (July 1996).*

Clinical Features of Fibromyalgia

Ninety percent of patients experienced the following symptoms:

- Generalized pain
- Fatigue
- Stiffness
- Morning fatigue

Seventy to ninety percent of patients experienced the following symptoms:

- Post-exertional malaise
- Sleep disturbances
- Morning stiffness
- Headaches
- Tenderness
- Swollen feeling in tissues
- Numbness and tingling
- Cognitive impairment (e.g., decreased memory and concentration)
- Dizziness
- Sensitivity to noise, smells, and stress
- Menstrual cramping
- Dry mouth

Fifty to seventy percent of patients experienced the following symptoms:

- Irritable Bowel Syndrome
- Blurred vision
- Mood swings
- Heart palpitations
- Cold extremities
- Feverous feeling
- Allergies

Fifteen to fifty percent of patients experienced the following symptoms:

- Restless legs
- Muscle twitches
- Itchy skin
- Hearing disturbances (e.g., tinnitus)

- Night sweats
- Migraines
- Breathing problems
- Infection proneness
- Skin problems (e.g., rashes)
- Multiple chemical sensitivities

Less than fifteen percent of patients experienced:
- Major depression (concurrent)

Please note that these symptoms are not diagnostic criteria for a diagnosis of fibromyalgia. These are descriptions of symptoms based on a survey of fifteen hundred of Dr. Olin's patients (Olin, 1996).

Unfortunately, scientists and doctors have not been able to find a single mechanism to explain the widespread pain that fibromyalgia sufferers experience. No one has been able to sort out why many of the additional symptoms are also present. Research has been continuing around the world to try to find causes of fibromyalgia and better treatments. Dr. Mark Pellegrino (who will be discussed in Part Three of Book Three) notes in his book *Understanding Post-traumatic Fibromyalgia* (1996) that a variety of factors may be important. These factors include genetics, trauma, altered nerve and muscle patterns, infectious disorders, abnormal sleep patterns, neurotransmitter and endocrine abnormalities, immune system disorders, and possibly allergic factors (page 3).

Not only is fibromyalgia a painful and often disabling illness, it is also complicated. Yet, there is no doubt that scientists are getting much closer to discovering the physical and medical basis of fibromyalgia. In a recent review, new findings from diagnostic imaging studies, clinical studies looking for biological makers in the brain and spinal cord, and studies of sleep deprivation, pain and cognitive impairment have shown much promise (Sumptom and Moulin, 2008).

Fibromyalgia is not a new illness. Scientists and doctors have known about this condition for many years. In fact, there are references to its description as far back as 1816 by Dr. William Balfour, a surgeon at the University of Edinburgh in Scotland. Later in 1904, Dr. Gowers described an illness he called "fibrositis," which he believed to be a pain disorder caused by damage to the fibrous tissue of the muscle. Groundbreaking research was done by Dr. Smythe and Dr. Moldofsky, in the mid-1970s. They led the charge toward a new understanding of fibromyalgia. Their findings established a connection between widespread aches, pains, fatigue, and patterns of sleep disturbance recorded in the sleep laboratory. Later research confirmed that both long-term pain and poor sleep are core symptoms of fibromyalgia (Pellegrino, 1996; Starlanyl and Copeland, 1996, 2001).

The stage was set, then, for a large multicenter study sponsored by the American College of Rheumatology. Results from this large study led to the establishment of formal diagnostic criteria, now accepted throughout the world. In 1987, the American Medical Association recognized fibromyalgia as a true illness and a major cause of disability (Starlanyl and Copeland, 1996, 2001). Then, an official definition of fibromyalgia was detailed in the Copenhagen Declaration at the Second World Congress on Myofascial Pain and Fibromyalgia in August 1992. This definition was accepted by the World Health Organization, January 1, 1993. Fibromyalgia was described here as "the presence of unexplained widespread pain, aching, persistent fatigue, generalized morning stiffness, non-refreshing sleep, and multiple tender points." Since then, both the International Association for the Study of Pain and the National Institute of Health in the United States have formally recognized fibromyalgia as a legitimate illness (Moldofsky and Merskey, 2005).

Fibromyalgia is usually diagnosed by specialists in rheumatology and often by specialists in physical medicine. Other medical specialists with an interest in pain and fibromyalgia may also diagnose this problem. Clinical and scientific studies have been able to clarify that fibromyalgia is not a psychiatric disorder. In his keynote speech, Dr. Olin stated that fibromyalgia is neither a psychosomatic disorder, nor is it a form of depression, an accident neurosis, or a malingering behavior (Olin, 1996). In fact, the Copenhagen Declaration stated that although depression and anxiety are common in people with fibromyalgia, these symptoms are likely caused by the physical condition itself. This is also true for the many other causes of chronic pain (Merskey, 2005).

• • •

Ashley suffered from neck and right-arm pain after her car accident. For several years, her sleep was broken, making it all the harder for her to cope with her pain. She became worn down, exhausted, and depleted of almost all energy. Additional pains started up in her back, hips, and knees.

After about three years, Ashley was diagnosed with fibromyalgia by a rheumatologist. This diagnosis finally explained her symptoms and helped to reduce her fears. She had worried, as do many people with unexplained symptoms, that maybe she was going crazy. This was not the case, of course, since many of Ashley's anxieties and frustrations settled down once her symptoms were explained to her. The explanation and diagnosis of fibromyalgia made sense to her and fit well with her widespread pain, fatigue, insomnia, and bowel problems.

Having this diagnosis reduced Ashley's confusion and some of the stresses that followed from her accident and injuries. Like others with chronic pain, there were many losses and life changes that her pain and limitations had forced upon her. Like Suzanne, Mike, and Sarah, she began the long road to recovery by regaining control over her chronic neck and arm pain, her fibromyalgia pain symptoms, and the many related stresses in her life. In the following book, you will learn how Ashley and her new friends were able to make this approach work for them.

Book Two

HEALING AND RECOVERY

Part One:
Highlights from Ashley's Journal

We all wanted this pain program to work out. It was a grueling time for us; we all pushed hard just to survive. It was the longest six weeks of my life.

As I look back, I can see Ashley was the real keener. As she unpacked on that first day, I noticed a pretty, fabric-covered journal that was to be her constant companion throughout her stay in hospital. She took this notebook everywhere – to all her appointments, treatment sessions, family meetings, and even to our late-night gatherings in Mike's room.

I had a chance to look at some of Ashley's notes one day. They were incredibly detailed, with material from readings, doctor's appointments, group treatment sessions, as well as from the many discussions between the four of us. Some of her thoughts and ideas really hit home with me. I asked Ashley if I could share some of her writings with other people who were in pain. She was flattered and readily agreed. Here are some of the highlights from Ashley's journal and a few stray thoughts of my own.

Suzanne

CHAPTER ONE

Pain and Chronic Pain

Two Main Types of Pain

Short-term pain is different from long-term pain. Both are physical. Both are real. Both can lead to a lot of suffering.

Most of you know something about short-term pain. You may have experienced pain from a cut, a burn, surgery, a toothache, or childbirth, as examples. Short-term pain can range from mild to severe. It can be unbearable while it lasts. Suzanne knew a lot about short-term pain as a dentist and as a patient. She had a surgical operation without anesthesia or pain medication and was able to control the severe short-term pain. It was amazing to hear her tell us how she did it.

With short-term pain, there is always an end in sight. With treatment or time, you know that it will be temporary. Each hour of each day, the pain gets a little better. This helps you to maintain hope and strength. You know it will soon be over.

Chronic pain is very different; it is more like a never-ending endurance test. It will not soon be over. You struggle to survive and to hang on to whatever hope you can. You try to conserve your strength so that you can last another day. Suzanne had much more difficulty with her chronic neck and back pain than she did pain from her surgery. The surgical pain was more intense, but it did not last that long. Hours compared to years; it was no contest.

Escalations of Pain

Temporary escalations in pain are called flare-ups. Pain can flare up just like a fire can. Imagine how the intensity of a fire increases when you blow on it. Now imagine pouring gas on the fire. This is what happens during a flare-up, especially a bad one.

Flare-ups can last for a few minutes or for weeks on end. Often, they involve severe pain and can be harder to cope with than the constant background pain. Even though they are short-term in nature, flare-ups can feel like they will never end. They can be very convincing.

Sometimes flare-ups can build on top of each other. This happens when a new flare-up is triggered before the last one has had a chance to settle down. Back to back flare-ups can be especially difficult. There is no time to recover from one flare-up before the next one sets in. These are times when pain can really become overwhelming.

The four of us spent a lot of time in the hospital program learning about our own flare-ups. We had to try and sort out the activities and stresses that could trigger a flare-up, as well as figure out a recovery plan for the flare-ups that were unavoidable. Sometimes, weather changes can trigger unavoidable flare-ups, for instance. Fortunately, many flare-ups can be avoided. We learned a lot of very useful strategies by studying the patterns and details of our pain flare-ups. This was a good start to learning some real pain control.

Flare-ups and Chain Reactions

Sometimes flare-ups are simple. You move the wrong way, get a sharp pain in your neck, and it takes an hour or so for it to settle down. At other times, flare-ups can work like a chain reaction. Here is an example. Pain interferes and reduces your sleep. Your pain is worse the next day. Now that your pain is stronger, it interferes even more with your sleep the next night, leading to even higher pain levels the following day. In this simple example, there are only two elements to the chain reaction – pain and sleep. They keep aggravating each other, as your pain increases and your sleep decreases. Then you "crash" for several days, resting in bed trying to recover.

Complicated chain reactions can encompass many parts of your life. A chain reaction can start with an injury, then lead to prolonged pain, loss of work, loss of benefits, big financial stresses, insomnia, despair, and then escalate to even higher levels of pain. If you are not able to return to work or have your benefits restored, higher pain levels can last for years. This mountain of pain can overpower almost anyone and make recovery very difficult.

Sarah had a lot of experience with this type of chain reaction. After her car accident, she was battling with many of these stresses. Her pain symptoms were flared up for several years. It was only after she started working with Evelyn that her stresses and pain began to lessen. This was a blessing for her.

Mountains of Pain to Climb

Pain can build in intensity and keep building hour-by-hour, day-by-day. This happens most often when your injury or illness is aggravated by repeated activities. This repeated aggravation was occurring with Sarah. Even after she learned to settle her pain down with relaxation, she would jump back into gardening or house cleaning. This burst of activity would send her back pain soaring again. If the aggravation continues, then your pain will keep building and building, with each day bringing higher levels of pain.

Pain can also escalate following nights of poor sleep and daytime exhaustion, especially if this pattern continues day after day. These factors can directly aggravate your injuries and trigger increases in pain. Pain can also build up when you become weakened with prolonged stress. Sarah was trapped in a long war with her insurance company. Mike was fighting workers' compensation, although his battles were less intense than Sarah's. At least he was receiving regular benefits. These situations can be horrible binds for people with chronic pain. Not only do you have to deal with the stress and conflict, but you also try and survive the mountain of pain that has built up.

CHAPTER TWO

The Impact of Chronic Pain

Chronic Pain Is More than Just Pain

This was a very new idea to me and I think to all of us. We found out that the whole chronic pain program was based on this idea. This simple phrase says a lot: chronic pain is more than just pain.

In the hospital program, we learned chronic pain is long-term pain that gathers additional components over time. These parts include the pain symptoms themselves, of course. For many people, several parts of their body are in pain at the same time. (This is especially true for people with fibromyalgia.) Other components include the limitations caused by pain symptoms and their physical causes, insomnia, fatigue, and the many ways all these parts can affect your mood, personality, relationships, and life.

Chronic pain can change people's lives. It can lead to serious losses of work, financial security, personal relationships, and even marriages and families. These changes can build up over time. Chronic pain is not just pain; it is all these pieces added together. Our pain program helped us to see this big picture. When we could see how our injuries, our pains, and our changed lives were affecting each other, it all made perfect sense. This big picture allowed us to think about healing and recovery in a whole new way.

Pain Can Trigger Anger and Powerlessness

Relentless back and leg pain made Sarah feel angry and powerless, as did her physical limitations. We all knew what this felt like, but Sarah was really having a difficult time with all of this.

Sarah was quite limited by her back and leg injuries. It was very hard for her to accept and cope with these limitations. She would try to fight back and force her injured body to do more than it could. As she fought, her pain kept building until she had no choice but to stop. This pattern repeated over and over again, which in turn, made her feel angry, powerless, and very depressed.

She hated being out of work. She hated to be dependent on others to help her. She hated being hounded by her insurance adjuster and felt she had no power to get this adjuster out of her life. She felt trapped, which made these feelings all the stronger.

I am glad Sarah met Evelyn. This was a definite turning point for her. Evelyn showed her how to direct all this intense emotion toward activities that would help with her recovery. We were all amazed at how well it worked. Evelyn really did help save Sarah's life.

Chronic Pain Can Change Lives

Over time, chronic pain can seep into every corner of your life. Injuries and illness can affect your health. They can damage a particular part of your body, such as your back and neck. Long-term pain also puts an enormous physical strain on your whole bodily system – your immune system, your heart, your emotions, your sleep cycle, and your blood pressure.

It doesn't stop there. Long-term pain can bring limitations that interfere with work or caring for your family. Relentless pain can make you irritable and hard to live with. Sarah found this out the hard way. Her marriage eventually broke down under the strain.

It would be hard to find an area of life that is not affected by long-term pain. This was certainly true for all of us. It was somewhat depressing to be faced with these facts, to tell the truth. Our hospital program was reality therapy with no holding back. Seeing the seriousness of our injuries and our damaged lives jolted us into really committing to a plan of recovery.

You Do Not Want to Go to War with Your Pain

When you go to war with pain, pain always wins. This was a very difficult lesson for all of us to learn. The harder you fight, the stronger your pain becomes. It is like trying to fight fire with gasoline. You just end up getting burned.

When you fight back, your emotions escalate and become more intense. This triggers stress and changes in your body and brain. Your brain produces more adrenaline and a variety of hormone changes. These all serve to increase your pain levels and aggravate the injured parts of your body.

Intense emotions can make you stronger, temporarily. Over time, though, day after day, intense emotions can weaken you and wear you down. Your energy to control your pain runs out. There is less of you left over. When you are out of gas, you are stuck. It is very hard at this point to pick yourself up and start moving forward again.

Going to war with pain can only lead to more pain, more limitations, and more losses. This was one of the most important lessons I learned in the chronic pain program; it is a lesson I will never forget.

CHAPTER THREE

Hidden Keys to Control

Why Fighting Can Feel Like the Only Way

There is no doubt pain causes you to suffer and urges you to fight back. It can truly feel like you have no choice but to react through battle. But how could you possibly win a war against yourself, against your injured body?

Sarah wasn't the only one caught in this trap. For a long time, Mike tried to push himself at the gym as a way to recover from his shoulder injury. He could not accept the limitations this injury had caused. His experiences of the past taught him that exercise and strengthening often helped with his sports injuries. When this approach did not solve his chronic shoulder pain, his first attempts were to push even harder and fight back with a fury. Day after day, he would try to increase the number of repetitions for each of his exercises and increase the weights he was using. He became a desperate man. It took him quite a while to realize his shoulder was not only becoming more painful with repeated flare-ups, but was actually getting weaker. Mike was finally forced to give up these desperate attempts. Exercise is still important. Mike learned that exercise must be incorporated in a reasonable and balanced way – it must become part of his life, not reduced to a daily battle.

Fighting may feel like the only way, but it is not. Planned, patient, and well-thought-out approaches are what really work.

Pain Control Is Not Black or White

Imagine trying to drive your car if you only had two options – full brake or full gas. You wouldn't get very far. You certainly would have little or no real control over the car. Pain control works in a similar way. It is not something that is black or white, full on or full off. It is in the gray areas, the details, where real control happens.

Sometimes taking one-half or one-quarter of a pain pill works better than taking a whole pill*. Sometimes a twenty-minute break works better than pushing until you can't go any further, requiring a full sleep. It takes a little calmness and composure to think this way. This was a tough idea for Mike to embrace, but one that really paid off for him in the end.

* Your physician can tell you which medications can be split safely and which ones cannot.

Avoidance Does Not Bring Control

Awareness does

In fact, this was the central message behind Suzanne's story of her surgery. Her control over pain was unbelievable. She didn't try to avoid the pain from surgery; she became more aware of it. She paid attention to the details of how she felt, what was going on in her body, and what the surgeon was doing to her. Fighting the pain, or trying to push it away, would only have made the pain stronger and harder to manage. It would also have weakened her.

Without awareness of your pain, its patterns and flare-ups, you will have little chance of learning ways to control it. Listening to your body, paying attention to its ups and downs, and working with it really pays off in the long run. Besides, it is tough to run away from your own body – practically impossible, I would say. Paying more attention allows you to be kinder and gentler to your injured body, which really does need your help.

Tracking Down the Triggers

To obtain lasting relief, you need to find ways to reduce all the things that can aggravate your pain – or at least as many of them as possible. This means tracking down the triggers that can set off pain flare-ups and cause a setback.

We learned about many of the common triggers in our hospital program. Lack of sleep, over-activity, and intense stress are the most common triggers experienced by almost all people with long-term pain. We knew these triggers well.

I also had my own triggers. I was frightened of letting down my husband and parents. When I couldn't do as much around our home, I was worried this would upset my husband. Sometimes our home was a mess, especially after a big flare-up would put me to bed for two to three days. Sometimes I was grouchy and wanted to be alone. What kind of wife was I being then? My husband and I have spent many hours talking about my fears and stresses. This really helped. I have learned to understand and be more realistic about my worries. Talking doesn't take them all away, but my worries are a lot less intense now. My husband also helped me to pinpoint some of the other stresses that would trigger increased pain. Having a compassionate observer living with you each day can really help. Having a real partner is a blessing.

Control Over Pain and Life

In addition to pain, injuries and illnesses can bring losses and disruption to your life. Many changes can be suddenly forced upon you and your family. These changes can bring high levels of stress and interfere with your healing and recovery.

If your pain is short-term, disruption to your life will usually be temporary. As soon as you feel better, you can go about putting your life back together. Long-term pain brings greater disruption to a situation that will not get better on its own. Mending your life will require work, just as managing your pain will require effort. The most successful recoveries come when individuals try to reduce the stresses that can aggravate their injuries and pain and try to regain some control in their lives.

Regaining control is important for every area of your body and your life. Who would have thought that dating would have helped Mike so much? He used the imagery and relaxation exercises to increase his self-esteem and confidence. This helped him to be less fearful of relationships, to start dating again, and to eventually meet his new girlfriend. He is now less stressed, has fewer flare-ups, and has more energy that he can use to focus on his recovery.

Increased control over pain *and increased control over your life* go hand-in-hand to produce the best results.

CHAPTER FOUR

Hidden Keys to Healing

Your Body Is Not Your Enemy

Although it may seem like your body is working against you when you are really hurting, your injured body is not your enemy. Your body is hurt. It needs to be cared for and strengthened, not fought against, not hurt more.

Even at the gym, your goal is not to attack your body. You do not want to punish it, especially when it has already been weakened by injury or illness. Instead, you want to work with your body and your injuries. You want to nurture them. You want to strengthen the injured parts of your body and your body as a whole. This will help you to avoid serious flare-ups and to help keep your energy up. These efforts will give the best results, as you and your body both work together.

After I became pregnant, my family doctor gave me a gentle, but serious wake-up call. He did not want me to overexert myself. He did not want me suffering flare-up after flare-up. He knew that pain flare-ups would weaken me and make it more difficult for my body to care for the baby growing inside of me. This did wake me. Now, more than ever, it was important for me to work with my injuries, my body, and my growing child. My pain symptoms responded, with lower levels of pain and fewer flare-ups. I also gained some much needed energy.

Fear of Pain Can Trigger More Pain

Sometimes fear and panic can send you spinning. These intense emotions can also trigger flare-ups of pain. This is true even when it is the pain itself that frightens you.

Fear of pain seems to come in two basic varieties. One is a fear that your pain will never end. Individuals experience this fear mostly at times when their pain is very strong. When you look closely, you can see that this fear of pain is really a fear that the strong pain will never end. Usually this strong pain is due to a flare-up. It feels as though the pain will never end – most intense pain does feel this way. Flare-ups will usually settle, though, if time is given to heal.

This is very important to remember. Flare-ups are temporary; they do settle. Your pain will calm down, just as it has all the other times. A necessary part of controlling pain is to control your fear of pain.

Panic Flare-ups

The second type of pain fear is more of a panic. It also occurs when pain levels are highest.

This type is a fear that the pain will keep escalating and escalating to the point where you lose all composure and control. Sometimes people in this situation also fear they will go crazy, although this would be very rare. When this panic sets in, it can be a real crisis. The escalating pain triggers panic. The panic is very powerful, very stressful, and sets off a chain reaction, leading to even higher levels of pain. The pain and panic keep aggravating each other, making it difficult for either one to settle down.

When this happens, you need help to reassure you this is a temporary situation. This help may come from someone close to you, or your doctor. You may need pain medication to stop the escalating cycle. For some people, anti-anxiety medication can decrease the panic and help the flare-up to settle down. For others, the combined pain and panic flare-up can be so exhausting, they eventually collapse in bed. A much needed rest will usually help greatly in settling down both the pain and the panic. This situation provides a vivid illustration of how pain and stress work together, almost trying to top each other as they torture you.

You Can't Get Better, Until You Stop Getting Worse

What could be simpler than that?

In theory, it is simple. In practice, it is often very difficult. Yet, your recovery depends on it.

In the first months after your injury, you try to fight back and not give in to the pain. As your pain continues past the time you thought it should have been resolved, you may become frightened and push harder. But, if you push too hard, too often, your flare-ups will never have a chance to settle down. You will have more pain and be more limited. How can you get better under these conditions?

This is a message we heard over and over again in our chronic pain program. And, believe me, it took a while to sink in. One of our counselors compared our struggle to those of long-distance runners. If they push too hard, too often, they will use up all their energy, burn out, and never finish the race. To be a successful distance runner, one needs to learn when to slow down, when to speed up and, most importantly, how to keep going. What takes time to learn is how to minimize the pain flare-ups that make it so hard to keep going and keep moving forward. Living with long-term pain requires not only a marathon of endurance, but also a marathon of hope.

Finding Your Self-Worth Again

With long-term pain and physical limitations, your self-esteem can take a beating. It is hard to feel good about yourself when you can't do the things you need to do.

Imagine playing golf with a sore neck or back. If the pain is not too bad, it can be done. Golf is not as physically demanding as compared to some other sports. But, you may not be able to play as well. Your enjoyment of the game may suffer if your scores get too high or your pain increases too much.

It is necessary to find some non-physical ways to enjoy your life and to help you feel good about yourself again. Sometimes more social activities can help. Learning new skills works for many people. This is a huge change, especially for people whose life and identity have been devoted to physical interests and activities. The payoff can be well worth the change, with less stress, less pain, and more of a life.

Give yourself a chance. You're worth it.

CHAPTER FIVE

Picking Yourself Up

Thank you for your patience and continuing interest. I know it is difficult to concentrate, page after page, with all the pain attacking you. Reading has been especially hard after my injuries started. It used to be so easy.

The past chapters of Book Two have been drawn from Ashley's notebook. We were all so lucky to have her notes to help us. The next few chapters are mostly my ideas though. Ashley inspired me to add a few of my own thoughts and observations. I hope they can help you.

Suzanne

First, Stop Falling

It is very hard to move forward toward recovery when you are still falling backward. Yet, without any solid footing, you cannot stop the falling. This can happen when you get injured, can't work, can't keep up with your bills, and can't stop falling behind financially. Recovery and healing are almost impossible with such powerful forces pressing down on you.

A first step toward recovery is securing some type of solid financial footing. You need to make sure you receive all the income replacement benefits that are legally available to you. This is necessary to protect you and your family. It is also necessary to protect yourself from the overwhelming stresses that can send your pain levels soaring and interfere with any type of treatment or recovery.

Safety first. Security first. Then healing and recovery will have a fighting chance.

Uncertainties Can Hold You Back

Losses can set you back and keep you falling. They certainly did for me. Uncertainties are stressful, too, but less so. They can keep you treading water, tire you out, and interfere with any kind of forward movement or recovery.

Of course, after serious or prolonged injury, there are many uncertainties in your life. Many questions arise. When will the pain go away? Why can't my doctors fix my injuries? What happens if I can't go back to work? How will I support my family? These questions can haunt you. I know because they sure haunted me. They haunted all of us.

As you can tell from this journal, Ashley is a note taker and list maker. That is how she gets through life. After she was injured, it became her lifeline. She wrote out questions before each meeting with her doctors and therapists. She wrote down the answers they gave. Often this triggered more questions, which she wrote down for the next meeting. She learned some things and gradually felt less uncertain about her injuries and future. For some questions, she was never able to get any clear answers – even years later. Maybe the answers to these questions have not been discovered yet, such as when a cure will be found for chronic pain. They are still in her notebook, though. And one by one, she is getting rid of the many uncertainties that hold her back. Uncertainties make her feel hesitant and weak. She wants to feel strong and confident again. Her notebook helps. It has helped all four of us.

A Verdict Is No Cure

Some doctors, lawyers, insurance adjusters, and everyday citizens still believe that once your lawsuit is over you will be cured. Your pains will magically disappear and you can return to work and a normal life. Wouldn't this be nice?

Life doesn't work out this way, though, and never has. Scientists have studied this issue in numerous research projects over the years. The findings have been quite clear. Chronic pain does not end when your case is settled. Your life may be less stressful because the insurance companies and lawyers are out of your life. With less stress, your pain may lessen. For this reason, it is very helpful to have your dealings with insurance companies end as soon as possible. But settlements and court victories, however useful in paying your debts, cannot cure chronic pain.

A verdict is no cure.

Searching for a Cure

We were all searching and hoping – and praying – each time we visited a new doctor or tried a new treatment. I was even hopeful when I had to visit insurance doctors.

A physiotherapist once tried to convince me that a cure was never going to happen. That really depressed me. I don't think he meant to get me so down. He just wanted me to be able to focus on my stretching and exercises and to get as strong as I could, even with my pain. He told me that some patients get stuck in their search for a cure. They put their lives on hold until the next doctor's visit, or the one after that. Years can go by this way, and if patients are not working to get stronger, he said, they could grow weaker and even more limited.

I know I have not given up hope. I am always checking out new research at the library and on the Internet. This helps me realize just how much pain research is conducted all over the world. I am always asking my doctors if they have read or heard about anything new. I like to share these new findings whenever I can, with whoever will listen. I make copies and take them to my doctors and therapists. They tell me that they like to have all the new information available, then share it with their coworkers. Maybe some day, I can put this stuff together in a book and share it with the millions of other people that live each day in pain.

This does not mean that I am stuck in a search for a cure. I have not put my treatments or recovery on hold.

For me, working on getting better and still having hope, go hand-in-hand. It all helps me to get stronger. I was watching Dr. Phil one day, and he said it well: It is okay to pray, but don't stop rowing for shore.

Success Can Lift You Up

While pain and loss can run you down, success can lift you up. Even minor successes can boost your energy reserves and make you feel like you are worth something again.

These successes can include improvements in your physiotherapy routines, helping others in your volunteer work, earning a good grade in the schooling you return to, or succeeding in the part-time work you just started. I was able to get a huge boost by succeeding in my return to part-time work. It was only for a few hours a week and I had to pay all my earnings back to the insurance company. (That part was just wrong.) I couldn't do regular dentistry work, even part-time. This was very hard to swallow. It still is. But, the opportunity to do some training and supervising at the dental school turned out to be a big success for me. I stopped sinking, and started to experience less stress and fewer flare-ups. I have not looked back since.

Sometimes, successes are hard to come by for people in pain. But, when they come, they sure do help.

CHAPTER SIX

Faster Roads to Recovery

This is still me – again. I think I have taken over Ashley's journal. I can't help myself. These ideas, even my own, get me excited and I want to share them. Please bear with me.

This is Suzanna on a roll.

Priorities and Recovery

For people in pain, there is no greater priority than pain relief, and if possible, permanent pain relief. You want your pain to go away, before you have to start putting your disrupted life back together. It makes perfect sense, really. Pain is the source of your suffering. If your injuries can be cured, you can go back to your old life and not have to worry about making any changes.

This was Ashley's plan before she entered the chronic pain program. To tell the truth, she was hoping for a miracle. She thought this program would cure her painful injuries. After this "miracle" happened, she and her husband would start a family. Actually, starting a family was her plan even before enrolling in the program. With each new doctor – and there were many – she became more hopeful, even desperate, for a cure. She was still hoping and searching for a cure by the time she ended up in the chronic pain program. By then, however, three years had passed.

Her friends in the program and her family doctor all helped her to realize that if she was waiting for a cure, she might have to wait forever. If she wanted to have a child, it was now or never.

In the year after the pain program, Ashley did become pregnant. She had many fears about not being able to carry and raise a child. But, at least one big stress had lifted. Surprisingly, she started to feel better, physically as well. It turned out that working on her pain management and her life management at the same time, succeeded in helping both parts. Now, she had a new life, and a family.

Moving Forward Instead of Fighting the Past

You have only so much energy. This supply of energy is decreased when you live in pain. Someone told me once that living with constant pain is like having the lights left on in your car, night after night. Your battery gets drained and it becomes harder and harder to recharge.

When your supplies are low, it is all the more important to be careful about how you spend the precious energy you have left. You have learned how fighting your pains and pushing yourself leads to flare-ups and higher levels of pain. Fighting also robs you of this precious energy. You need this energy to get through each day. This energy is needed to plan how to move forward in life and to make whatever changes are necessary, so that your life becomes more manageable. Recovery becomes possible when you learn to stop fighting your injured body and start moving forward, toward a new life.

This was a message we heard over and over in the hospital program. Sometimes, we became defensive and didn't want to hear it again, but the counselors were persistent. I am glad for this. It took a while, but I think the message finally sunk in for all of us – even bullheaded Sarah.

Freedom and Independence

Chronic pain can interfere with your life by forcing you to become more dependent on others. This can happen in many little ways, such as needing extra help with such things as household chores, childcare, or yard work.

If you are out of work, this dependence can infect you in a deeper way. Being out of work forces you to become dependent on financial benefits from others – an insurance company, workers' compensation, the government, or a company disability plan. This is a high pressure situation to be in. You never feel like your life is your own. It knocked me down and nearly killed Sarah.

If you are able to work, now or in the future, do everything possible to make this happen. This may include working modified or lighter duties, changing jobs, or even retraining. Mike found out from his rehab psychologist that his workers' compensation company would even pay for him to go to school and learn a new career. Some people are offered buyouts from their insurance company. This may be an option if you are too injured to return to work. Whatever way you can, try to get the insurance system out of your life. You will have less stress, more freedom and independence, and more energy to focus on recovery. Your body will also thank you.

Sometimes Change Is Necessary

Change is hard for most people, even a small change. Change forced upon you by injury and loss can be even more overwhelming. Having to change your career because of limitations and pain is one of the toughest obstacles on the road to recovery.

Most people are in their current jobs or career for good reasons: good pay, enjoyable work, security, and a network of friends at work. The thought of having to give up these benefits and move to an unfamiliar job can seem threatening and unimaginable. This is how Mike felt when he had to give up his construction job. He found out, though, that there was help for him during this transition, through his workers' compensation plan. His schooling was paid for. His benefits continued while he was in school and during his job search, once school was finished. There was a back-up pension available to him, if his future job ended up paying him less than his old job.

Even with all this retraining and financial help, it took a while for Mike to take this step. He always felt he was forced into it and couldn't help becoming defensive. This was a normal human reaction to forced change. With help from his rehab psychologist and compensation caseworker, Mike was able to make it happen. He had no regrets.

If change is necessary for you, there may be more help and support for you than you realize. Talk with your lawyer, your doctors, and anybody that may help. Your insurance company will often not volunteer this information, but with a little digging, you can usually find out what might be possible and worth fighting for.

Your Comeback Story

I heard an idea one day from a very dynamic woman I met at physiotherapy. Cory was once a career counselor who worked helping managers and executives find new jobs after they had been laid off. These managers were embarrassed by having to look for new jobs and hated being asked the same questions over and over again, by friends, family, or whoever heard they were out of work. To cope with these questions, one manager developed a short story to tell people whenever this situation came up. He called it his thirty-second commercial. My friend at the support group liked this idea so much, she adapted it to help her deal with the endless questions about her injuries. Cory called her version her Comeback Story.

Cory's comeback story had four basic parts: the past, her accident, her rehabilitation, and a happy ending. The past included a couple of details about her former work. Then she mentioned she was in a car accident several years ago and suffered from painful neck and back injuries. Next, she purposely talks briefly about how much her doctors and therapists have helped her. Some have helped more than others, but Cory describes it this way to avoid all the "why aren't your doctors doing more?" questions. These "why" questions can be very difficult and are too depressing to explain. Finally, in her happy ending, she notes she is doing pretty well, still seeing her doctors, getting stronger each day, and hoping to return to work one day. Then, without taking a breath, she changes the subject to focus more on the other person.

I have started fine-tuning my own comeback story. It really helps me navigate all the times when I am stuck having to explain myself. I hate being in this position, but, short of being rude, it is hard to avoid. Thankfully, I have my comeback story whenever I need it.

CHAPTER SEVEN

Seven Simple Truths About Chronic Pain

Seven Simple Truths

One Chronic pain is real, not imagined. It is never "all in your head."

Two You can't get better until you stop getting worse. The first step is to recognize this pattern. Even by itself, this step can make a big difference.

Three When you go to war with pain, pain always wins. There are much better ways to gain control over your pain.

Four A simple flare-up formula: pain causes stress, which then causes more pain. If not stopped, the flare-up keeps building to a mountain of pain. The best way to decrease a flare-up is by reducing the aggravations that are feeding the fire.

Five For some people, coping with constant background pain is the easier part. Repeated flare-ups are what bring you down. Reducing flare-ups (and learning to avoid as many as you can) are the best ways to gain pain control and a speedy recovery.

Six If your benefits are cut off, recovery is over. When your losses escalate, it is almost impossible to gain the energy, strength, and pain tolerances necessary to move forward in your life. Make sure you work with your doctors and lawyers to protect your benefits.

Seven Helplessness and anger can give pain the power to defeat you. They add fuel to the fire. But not all types of anger are harmful. Anger directed toward simple, achievable goals can give you a powerful boost toward recovery.

Part Two:

The True Story that Inspired Suzanne

CHAPTER ONE

A Tribute to Dr. Victor Rausch

Let me introduce the real hero of this story, Dr. Victor Rausch. Suzanne's story and experiences were modeled after Dr. Rausch's courage, skills, and achievements.

In 1978, Dr. Rausch underwent major abdominal surgery. He had his gallbladder removed without anesthesia or painkillers. This surgery was done in a city hospital by a team of surgeons and nurses. An anesthetist monitored Dr. Rausch's vital signs during surgery and was ready if an anesthetic became necessary. It never was. After a deep abdominal incision, his gallbladder was removed. This took a total of approximately seventy-five minutes for the surgery and stitches to be completed. Dr. Rausch described this process in a colorful way to author Robert Hercz: "They cut open your belly, open it up with clamps, and get in there and move your guts around" (Hercz, 2000, page 15).

After the surgery, Dr. Rausch was assisted off the operating table and was able to walk to the elevator and then to his room. Surgery took place on a Friday morning. Dr. Rausch recovered in hospital until the following Wednesday. The next Monday, Dr. Rausch was back at his dental office working. This was all documented in a 1980 article, published in a reputable scientific journal (Rausch, 1980).

Dr. Rausch accomplished this amazing feat with the use of self-hypnosis. He had been a student, practitioner, and teacher of hypnosis for many years. He spent five years in the Canadian Armed Forces, where he was able to study the powerful effects of hypnosis during extensive and painful dental surgeries. Later on, hypnosis was used in his dental practice. He has videotaped some of the complicated dental surgeries he performed on his patients. Hypnosis was used as the only anesthetic; no freezing or painkillers were administered.

Dr. Rausch also underwent a complicated dental operation, again without anesthesia or painkillers. On the videotape, one can see how Dr. Rausch calms himself with self-hypnosis. This dental surgery involved the removal of an impacted molar. Incisions were made in his gum. A flap was cut open. There was drilling of the bone to break up the large molar into pieces. It was necessary to dig out the molar and the nerve root. Stitches were inserted after the surgery was completed. Throughout this process, Dr. Rausch was able to communicate with the dental surgeon, even while under hypnosis and while controlling the pain. This did not seem to be a problem for him. He showed no signs of fear or stress. It was fascinating to watch his skills in action.

In many ways, Dr. Rausch's accomplishments are difficult to believe. It is not surprising that Mike, Ashley, and Sarah had such strong reactions to Suzanne when she told them the story of undergoing gallbladder surgery without anesthesia. Even for people who don't experience pain on a daily basis, it is hard to believe that anyone could undergo surgery without medication. Mike, Ashley, and Sarah knew all too well what it was like to live with serious levels of pain day-in and day-out. For them, Suzanne's story was beyond belief.

There is no doubt about the reality of Dr. Rausch's accomplishments. For people who really know what serious pain is like, however, his achievements are all the more remarkable. Dr. Rausch's gallbladder surgery is chronicled in the scientific article he published (Rausch, 1980), and Dr. Rausch's experiences and accomplishments are also described in an editorial written by Dr. Sheldon B. Cohen (1980).

Robert Hercz has written a brief lay description of Dr. Rausch, his surgery, and the growing popularity and uses of hypnosis. His article is entitled "Surgery Without Anesthetic: The Outer Limits of Hypnosis." It can be found in the magazine *Toronto Life* (2000).

Hypnosis has been a mysterious and often misunderstood phenomenon. In the following chapter, I have tried to relate hypnosis to experiences we all have in our day-to-day lives. Hypnosis is more common and ordinary than most people realize. However, the use of self-hypnosis as a replacement for anesthesia during surgery is not at all ordinary.

CHAPTER TWO

What Is Hypnosis?

Does hypnosis produce an out-of-the-ordinary, trance-like, "altered" state of consciousness? Dr. Irving Kirsch, from the University of Connecticut, and Dr. Steven Jay Lynn, from the University of Ohio, try to answer this fascinating question in an interesting and informative article published in the *American Psychologist* (Kirsch & Lynn, 1995).

Drs. Kirsch and Lynn discuss the growing acceptance of hypnosis as a helpful treatment for a wide variety of physical health problems, including pain. They also describe some of the controversies in this field. For instance, some doctors and scientists still believe that hypnosis involves an altered state of consciousness very different from a normal wakened state. It has been difficult for scientists to document this view, however. Despite many scientific investigations over the past fifty years, no clear evidence has been found for any physical differences in individuals when they are under hypnosis.

Researchers and clinicians still use the idea of "trance" to describe what is happening when people are under hypnosis. They describe this trance in more everyday terms. They argue that this altered state of trance is not necessarily unique to hypnosis, but can occur in different ways during ordinary individuals' everyday lives. Drs. Kirsch and Lynn offer some interesting quotes from researchers in the field to describe this everyday phenomenon.

As one example, Drs. Cheek and LeCron wrote:

> "At times everyone daydreams. This definitely is a trance state…Whenever we become absorbed in what we are doing, we slip into hypnosis…Any strong emotion may produce hypnosis. A state of shock, suddenly, is similar to a trance state." (p. 6)

Drs. Walters and Havens offer a similar description in their article from 1993:

> "The term trance refers to the day-dreamy state of mind often experienced by people when they meditate, listen to music, attend a long lecture, drive on a freeway at night, undergo a hypnotic induction, or wait patiently in a therapist's waiting room…Whether elicited by a hypnotist or induced by a long stretch of highway, a trance is a trance." (pp. 23–24).

Scientific research on hypnosis over the past twenty years has helped to knock down the many myths so popular in our society. Drs. Kirsch and Lynn provide a clear summary of the many things that hypnosis is not. It is now known that:

- The ability to experience hypnotic phenomena does not indicate gullibility or weakness.

- Hypnosis is not related to sleep.
- Hypnotic responsiveness depends more on the efforts and abilities of the person hypnotized than the skill of the hypnotist.
- Participants retain the ability to control their behavior during hypnosis. They are aware of their surroundings and can monitor events outside of themselves.
- Suggestions can be responded to with or without hypnosis, and the function of a hypnotic induction is merely to increase suggestibility to a minor degree.
- Hypnosis is not a dangerous procedure when practiced by qualified clinicians and researchers.
- Hypnosis does not increase the accuracy of memory. (Kirsch & Lynn, 1995)

The research evidence behind each of these ideas was summarized by Drs. Kirsch and Lynn in their 1995 article. Much has been learned about hypnosis from years and years of rigorous scientific research.

One of the more interesting points in this research is that participants can retain the ability to control their behavior during hypnosis and that they are aware of their surroundings. This was made very clear by Dr. Rausch as he described his experience of undergoing surgery without anesthesia. Suzanne's descriptions in Book One (*Unbelievable Pain Control*) also follow this idea. Of course, when an individual is performing the hypnosis himself, as did Dr. Rausch, who else would be in control?

There has been much intrigue over the years regarding what hypnosis actually is and what it is not. There have been numerous myths and sensational Hollywood stories about hypnosis. One can see from the points noted above just how many of these myths scientists have had to knock down. Suzanne wanted to avoid some of this mystery and intrigue as she described her experiences of undergoing surgery to her fellow patients in the chronic pain program. In her descriptions, she emphasized the practical exercises and techniques that she used. These were the standard techniques that Dr. Rausch used, including progressive muscle relaxation, dissociation, and rehearsal of the procedure in advance.

Dr. Cohen described an additional technique that Dr. Rausch used in his editorial description of Dr. Rausch's article (Cohen, 1980). He described how Dr. Rausch developed a strong awareness of the presence of one of the operating nurses and felt strengthened by his eye contact with her during the procedure. Suzanne wanted to emphasize this point as well to Sarah, Ashley, and Mike. She explained how she opened her eyes several times during the surgery and made eye contact with the surgeon. This helped to strengthen her as well as helping to reassure the surgeon that everything was going as planned.

Dr. Cohen gives an interesting anecdote in his editorial. In the above discussion, hypnosis was described as being a daydream-like trance. Dr. Cohen described an interview that was done with the famous violinist, Isaac Stern, from the Boston Pops series. He was asked whether he ever forgot what he was playing or where he was playing during a concert. He answered that his concentration and absorption were such that he really did not know, at times, where the stage that he was performing on was located. He was so absorbed in his music that he was not even sure what city he was in at the time. This degree of concentration and absorption is very similar to a hypnotic state. As another example, you may be driving home from work one day and realize that, as you pull into the driveway, you do not remember any of the trip you just completed. You did not remember stopping at the stop signs, making the turns that you did, which cars you were following or passing, or even what kind of buildings you passed along your route. This is an example of everyday absorption and an everyday hypnotic state. These everyday experiences are so familiar to us all – yet also quite fascinating.

But what is clinical hypnosis actually like? What happens when a doctor uses hypnosis to help lessen your pain? Below is a real-life hypnotic script used to help women reduce the pain and anxiety associated with a large core breast biopsy. In this procedure, a needle is inserted into a woman's breast to remove a piece of breast tissue. This tissue is later analyzed for the presence of cancerous cells. This hypnotic script appeared in an article published by Dr. Lang and her colleagues at the Beth Israel Deaconess Medical Center and Harvard Medical School (Lang et al., 2006). It is similar to most hypnotic procedures used in medical settings.

A Standardized Hypnotic Procedure

"We want you to help us help you learn a concentration exercise to help you get through the procedure more comfortably. It can be a way to help your body be more comfortable through the procedures and also deal with any discomfort that may come up during the procedure. It is just a form of concentration, like getting so caught up in a movie or a good book that you forget you are watching a movie or reading a book.

"Now what I want to do is to show you how you can use your imagination to enter a state of focused attention and physical relaxation. If you hear sounds or noises in the room, just use these to deepen your experience. Use only the suggestions that are helpful for you. There are a lot of ways to relax but here is one simple way:

> On one, I want you to do one thing – look up.
>
> On two, do two things – slowly close your eyes and take a deep breath.
>
> On three, do three things – breathe out, relax your eyes, and let your body float.

"That's good, just imagine your whole body floating, floating through the table, each breath deeper and easier. Right now, I want you to imagine you are floating somewhere safe and comfortable, in a bath, a lake, a hot tub, or just floating in space, each breath deeper and easier. Notice how with each breath you let a little more tension out of your body as you let your whole body float, safe and comfortable, each breath deeper and easier.

Good, now with your eyes closed and remaining in this state of concentration please describe for me how your body is feeling right now. Where do you imagine yourself being, what is it like? Can you smell the air? Can you see what is around you? Good, now this is your safe and pleasant place to be and you can use it in a sense to play a trick on the doctors. Your body has to be here, but you don't. So just spend your time being somewhere you would rather be.

"Now, if there is some discomfort, and there may be some with the procedure as they prepare you and give the anesthetic or insert the equipment, there is no point in fighting it. You can admit it, but then transform that sensation. If you feel some discomfort, you might find it helpful to make that part of your body feel warmer, as if you were in a bath. Or cooler, if that is more comfortable, as if you had ice or snow on that part of your body. This warmth and coolness becomes a protective filter between you and the pain.

"If you have any discomfort right now, imagine that you are applying a hot pack or you are putting snow or ice on it and see what it feels like. Develop the sense of warmth or cool tingling numbness to filter the hurt out of the pain.

"With each breath, breathe deeper and easier, your body is floating, filter the hurt out of the pain.

"Now again with your eyes closed and remaining in the state of concentration, describe what you are feeling right now."

If they are at their safe and comfortable place – reinforce it.

"What is it like now? What do you see around you? What are you doing?"

If they are in pain: "The pain is there but see if you can add coolness, more warmth, or make it lighter or heavier."

If no longer in pain: "Good, continue to focus on those sensations."

If still in pain: "You may want to focus on sensations in another part of your body. Now rub your fingertips together and notice all the delicate sensations in your fingertips and see how much you can observe about what it feels like to rub your thumb and forefingers together. How do you feel now?"

If not in pain: "Good, continue to focus on these sensations."

If still in pain: "Now imagine yourself being at ______________ (patient's safe place) where you said you felt relaxed and comfortable. What is it like now? What is the temperature? What do you see around you?"

If they state that they are worried: "Okay, your main job right now is to help your body feel comfortable, so we will talk about what is worrying you. But first, no matter what we discuss, concentrate on your body floating. So let's get the floating back into your body. Imagine you are in this favorite spot and when you are ready let me know by nodding your head and then we will talk about what is worrying you. But remember, no matter what we discuss, concentrate on your body floating and feel safe and comfortable. So what is worrying you?" (*Discuss*).

"How do you feel now?" *If not worried:* "Good, now continue to concentrate on your body floating, and feel safe and comfortable in your favorite place."

If after discussing patient has persistent worry, then: "Okay, picture in your mind a screen like a movie screen, TV screen, or a piece of clear blue sky. First picture a pleasant scene on it. Now picture a large piece of blue screen divided in half. All right, now on the left half, picture what you are worrying about on the screen. Now, on the right half, picture what you will do about it, or what you would recommend someone else to do about it. Keep your body floating, and if you are worrying about the outcome, okay, admit it to yourself, but your body does not have to get uptight about it. You may, but your body does not have to."

"Good, you know that whatever happens, there is always something you can do. But, for now, just concentrate on keeping your body floating and feeling safe and comfortable."

Sometimes throughout the procedure say: "If you feel any sense of discomfort, you are welcome to let me know about it. Use the filter to filter the hurt out of the pain, but by all means, let me know, and I will do what I can to help you with it as well. Whatever you do, just keep your body floating and concentrate on being in the place where you feel safe and comfortable."

When finished, say: "Okay, the procedure is over now. We are going to leave formally this state of concentration by counting backwards from three to one. On three get ready, on two with your eyes closed roll up your eyes and, on one, let your eyes open and take a deep breath and let it out. That will be the end of the formal exercise, but when you come out of it you will still have the feeling of comfort that you felt during it. Ready, three, two, one" (Lang et al., 2006).

• • •

Dr. David Spiegel, a well-known hypnosis researcher from the Stanford School of Medicine, wrote an editorial about Dr. Lang's work (Spiegel, 2006). He reviews the long historical roots and powerful effects of hypnosis. The article is not very long, but it is packed with fascinating details.

Thank you to Dr. Elvira Lang, and her associates at Beth Israel Deaconess Medical Center and Harvard Medical School, for permission to use the hypnosis script from their biopsy study.

Book Three

A CALL TO ACTION

Part One:

People Are Helping from Around the World

CHAPTER ONE

Sarah's New-Found Hope

Sarah had been angry for a long time. It was not just anger at the drunk driver, though.

The drunk driver who hit Sarah did enormous damage to her body and to her life. There was no doubt about that. Yet, her anger ran deeper and wider. Her insurance adjusters, who continued to deny both the necessary treatments for her injuries and her income replacement benefits, did additional damage. Her own insurance company kicked her when she was already down and kept kicking so she couldn't get up. These denials created a deep hurt in Sarah and became an important component of the severe depression that overpowered her. Having multiple sources of pain, depression, serious financial strain, and lack of treatment made coping and rehabilitation hard enough for Sarah. The additional stresses and rejections from her own insurance company made recovery almost impossible.

Sarah's recovery centered on finding a way to fight back. Sarah wanted relief from her back and leg pain, of course, which were the main sources of her suffering. She wanted to be less limited so she could return to work and a normal life. She hoped the chronic pain program would provide this relief. But, she also wanted to fight back against the injustices, the suffering, and the stress caused by the actions of her insurance company. To do this, she became involved with a group of pain sufferers and set up a Website to help others in pain. The purpose of this Website was to provide people in pain with the information and tools they needed to fight back in their own lives.

Sarah felt energized and inspired as she started to gather information for their Website. She found that the problems she experienced in getting treatment for her injuries were often the same as those experienced by other people in pain. There were many reasons for these obstacles. Some of these reasons involved misconceptions or ignorance among healthcare professionals regarding pain and its treatment. Sometimes professionals were worried about prescribing strong pain medications for fear of dependence or addiction. These fears made it difficult for these doctors to use the kind of medications that are often necessary to bring about relief for people in severe pain. Sometimes doctors did not have the time to obtain the education and training required in prescribing the necessary medications.

Sarah also found out that some of the obstacles were related to society's attitudes about pain. Powerful myths have continued in our society, even while the research on chronic pain has mushroomed. Some people still cling to the myth that chronic pain exists solely in the one's head, and the myth that people in pain are weak, fragile, and interested only in lawsuits. These kinds of myths can be found throughout all segments of society.

Sarah did not want to be bogged down in such negativity, though. She was well aware of the myths and misconceptions that can be found in healthcare providers, lawyers, insurance companies, employers, and even in society at large. What she wanted for her Website was new research and ideas that could really help people. She wanted her Website to instill some hope in the millions of people who are struggling with pain. Sarah found hope very hard to come by in her darkest days. But, she also knew the power of hope, as she tried to find the energy to cope with pain and to move her life forward.

Sarah wanted her Website to focus on uplifting examples of successful research and treatment in the chronic pain field. From her reading and researching, she found there was an enormous swell of activity devoted to helping treat people in pain and helping to advocate on their behalf. As she waded through Websites from pain societies, research organizations, and pain foundations, she found example after example of this great work. She could feel the sparks of hope ignite. She knew this would also help to give others a boost and help with some much needed validation.

Sarah organized the information and put these examples together, which are included in the chapters that follow. These examples help to make things more real for people in pain, she thought. As Sarah knew from her own experience, positive examples and real-life details were what helped to produce more lasting hope.

Please note: In the chapters that follow, there are many examples of Websites and connecting links to other Websites. These Websites can change frequently, with new information and links being added and updated. Sarah would often circle back every few weeks to her favorite sites, hoping to catch up with each new and exciting discovery.

CHAPTER TWO

A Decade of Pain Research and Control (2001–2010)

The United States Congress has declared the decade from 2001 to 2010 as the Decade of Pain Control and Research. In late 2000, the United States Congress passed into law a declaration that this ten-year period would be a decade devoted to helping people in pain. This was a unique opportunity for health organizations to increase the help they could offer to people in pain, in the United States, Canada, and around the world.

The American Pain Society, one of the leading organizations, set up a multi-year task force to get several projects underway for the Decade of Pain Control and Research. The society coordinated its activities with the American Pain Foundation, the American Academy of Pain Medicine, and the American Headache Society.

This task force set up four main areas of focus. These included research, professional awareness, public policy, and public awareness. They also worked with a nationally recognized public relations firm, Webber and Associates, to help publicize and promote their goals and activities. A Website was set up to help the public learn about all the activities that were being planned and implemented.

One of the most important goals for the Decade of Pain is to promote research on pain and pain treatments. Research was necessary to further understand the mechanisms behind the injuries and illnesses that cause pain. The goal here was to put pressure on funding agencies to allocate more money for research on pain, and more money into finding and developing new and more effective treatments.

The next step was to promote a greater awareness among professionals regarding the best ways to help people in pain. Many of the sponsored activities include educational campaigns, the development of pain courses at medical schools, specialty courses offered through conferences and healthcare organizations, and the development of a prestigious lecture series on pain. Increased training can keep doctors up-to-date and help them do even better work for people in pain.

The third goal was policy agenda. It is necessary to change government policies so that people with all types of pain can get the treatment they need.

The last main goal of this task force focused on public awareness. The purpose here was to increase the awareness of pain in the general public, and to increase funding dedicated toward the understanding and treatment of pain. Planned events included educational activities, a Decade of Pain Website, links to other Websites, the development of national and state pain awareness weeks, and the development of a special lecture series to be held in communities throughout the nation. An important element involves the development and distribution of pain-related educational materials for individuals and their families.

Sarah was caught off guard as she immersed herself in reading about the Decade of Pain. It was a pleasant surprise, though. Before she started setting up her own Website, she never heard of the Decade of Pain, yet, the organizers were already several years into it. She started reading about all the different agendas, the activities that were going on, and all the materials that were available for doctors and people in pain. She knew she was on the right track.

• • •

The Decade of Pain Website can be found at:
www.decadeofpain.org

CHAPTER THREE

Untying the Knot: The National Pain Awareness Campaign

The National Pain Foundation set up a joint project with the American Academy of Pain Medicine. This important campaign combines the efforts of the National Pain Foundation, which focuses on helping people in pain and the American Academy of Pain Medicine, which is an organization for pain-trained physicians. Together, patients and doctors have been able to accomplish a great deal with the *Untying the Knot* campaign.

Some of the goals of their National Pain Awareness Campaign are listed below:

- To increase the awareness of options for treating and managing pain
- To educate people in pain, their families, their health-care providers, the insurers, and others about new pain management procedures, medications, and devices
- To improve patient access to reliable pain care
- To educate the public about new innovations and progress in the field of pain medicine
- To involve the entire medical community in the support and promotion of pain awareness (National Pain Foundation; American Academy of Pain Medicine)

This pain awareness campaign goes about achieving these goals through a system of pain awareness ambassadors. So far, there have been over four hundred ambassadors who have registered. They are represented in every state in the United States and in twelve other countries. Educational materials, lectures, fact sheets, question and answer materials, and newsletters are all provided free of charge to these ambassadors, who then distribute this information and knowledge throughout each of the communities that they serve.

These two organizations are very serious about helping society to move forward and provide more awareness and better treatment for individuals in pain. As you can see from their Website (the Website address is found on the following page) there are a variety of materials provided free of charge, not only to the ambassadors, but also to the public. They even provide pre-written articles and editorials for ambassadors to send to their local newspapers for publication. There are also brochures that can be sent to healthcare providers and patients in the community. Strategies are offered for the development of partnerships between healthcare providers and groups that want to help each other and the community learn more about pain and help promote more effective treatments.

As Sarah read and researched about the National Pain Awareness Campaign, she realized this project hit upon her personal goals and also the goals for her Website. In her own way, Sarah became an ambassador for people in pain. This felt right as she realized this. She knew now this was an important step in helping her to overcome her anger and powerlessness. There are many ways to help others in pain, she thought, as well as to help in the move toward recovery. Sarah was on her way.

• • •

These Websites are full of helpful
and hopeful information:

National Pain Foundation:
www.nationalpainfoundation.org
For the *Untying the Knot* campaign see
National Pain Awareness link

American Academy of Pain Medicine:
www.painmed.org

CHAPTER FOUR

Your Own Pain Advocacy Program

The Pain Awareness Ambassador Program, as discussed in the previous chapter, is mainly one for healthcare professionals. The materials are mostly for trained professionals who can use these materials to educate the public and help other professionals learn about chronic pain and the new treatments available. This is an important role for professionals, since often they will be in a better position to help influence other professionals. But, pain advocacy is not just for professionals. There is too much to be done. We all need to help society, including insurers, to understand more about pain, so we can dispel the myths and misconceptions that often hurt and limit treatments and benefits for people in pain.

Sarah continued on her search and brightened when she came across a newsletter from the American Pain Foundation. This was a free newsletter called the *Pain Community News*. Inside were articles and examples of how individuals can become pain management advocates. The first part of the article entitled "Pain Management Advocacy: From the One to the Many" read: "It's the decade of pain control and research – it's time to take action and become a pain management advocate!" (Duersing, 2004)

The authors of the newsletter were calling on people to take action – especially people in pain, caregivers, and healthcare providers. These are the people who know how much work needs to be done.

An advocate is a supporter, a defender, a champion, and an activist. An advocate tries to educate people, to increase awareness, and to remove barriers. They help validate and give a voice to people in pain. When Sarah read this she knew she had landed in the right place. This newsletter was able to put into words what she wanted to do from the beginning of her Website project.

Lennie Duersing, the author of this article on pain management advocacy, presented a lot of very useful information. Not only did she provide a list of places and people to write to for more information, she was very clear in setting up some simple steps that each person could take on their own.

The first step is simple – to get informed. This involves learning as much as possible about pain, pain management, and local resources. She encouraged each person in pain to communicate their experiences with others. Personal experiences form the foundation for validating and supporting others. People in pain are not alone. Often, individuals are confused about their injuries and symptoms and do not feel confident in sharing their realities with others. The more you talk with other people in pain, however, the more you realize how much you have in common. This is an important bond and goes a long way toward supporting each other. It really starts with opening up and telling others what you know and what you have been through.

Lennie Duersing wants you to use your passion. "Pain is a serious problem and most likely, you will find that others have pain stories that they will want to share with you" (Duersing, 2004). This is the grassroots way to spread the word. It is effective and based on the truth of real life experiences.

This first step is what Duersing has called "personal advocacy" – helping people directly. There are many ways that you can help advocate with your experience, your knowledge, your energy, and your time. Duersing describes some of the ways that you can help.

You can spend time with others in pain, listening to them or helping them with some simple activities such as getting out to the store.

You can help people in pain with some of the skills that they may need to help them fight for themselves and to be active participants in their pain care.

You can help them by providing information about pain, about treatment options, and about where they can find help (Duersing, 2004).

As Lennie Duersing says, people with pain can be the most effective messengers. They can tell their stories, give support to others, speak at local events, give media interviews, and write to their legislators.

If you are a health professional treating people in pain, you can also help advocate at another level. Some of these ways involve:

Reassuring people that you are trying to understand their needs and will be there for them as much as you can.

Encouraging people in pain to be more active and to participate in their own care by learning about their condition, making their own decisions, and participating in pain support groups where possible.

You can help people in pain handle the many details involved in dealing with insurance and legal matters. These are important steps to helping others get the care and the support they need.

You can also encourage others to become pain advocates. You can help them gain some renewed purpose and energy in their lives as well as a new sense of empowerment.

For people in pain, caregivers, and healthcare professionals, one of the most important steps is to help promote the Pain Care Bill of Rights. This is a publication put out by the American Pain Foundation, and available from their Website. Feel free to make copies yourself and hand them out to other people you know in pain, your doctors, or any healthcare agency that can benefit.

Sarah has taken it upon herself to move up to the next step of pain advocacy. This is really a type of public awareness advocacy, which she is helping to make happen through her Website. She is not only reaching out to individuals on a one-to-one basis, but trying to educate the public. This includes providing materials through her Website directly to people in pain as well as to healthcare professionals, lawyers, insurance companies, and anyone who wishes to help ease the suffering for the millions of people who live each day in pain.

• • •

For more information refer to the
American Pain Foundation's Website at:
www.painfoundation.org

A free subscription to the *Pain Community News*
is also available from this Website, as is the
Pain Care Bill of Rights.

CHAPTER FIVE

Power over Pain: A Grassroots Movement

This amazing awareness campaign is expanding by leaps and bounds.

It's an exciting program called the Power over Pain program. Sponsored by the American Pain Foundation and the American Alliance of Cancer Pain Initiatives, it is a comprehensive public education campaign. The program is aimed at healthcare professionals, people in pain, and many other types of professionals and political decision-makers.

The Power over Pain program was launched by the North Florida Chapter of the American Society of Pain Management Nursing in 2002. This campaign has been so successful it has now been used in other states. The next states to set up programs were Connecticut, Kansas, Maryland, and Vermont. Each state received a grant, training, special materials for distribution, and assistance in organizing the campaign, to ensure its success.

The Power over Pain program was set up as an action-oriented public awareness and media campaign. The goals were to make effective pain management a healthcare priority at state and local levels. The public was provided with practical information about pain and its management. One of the goals was to help empower patients and families so that they can demand effective pain control. Another goal was to encourage healthcare professionals to make this new information about pain and treatment available to their patients.

If you want to become more actively involved, you can go to their Website and order a Power over Pain community action kit. This package includes a media guide as well as comprehensive how-to information for organizations that wish to put on their own public awareness campaigns. This kit also helps organizations with suggestions for building alliances with other interested groups, activity ideas, and strategies for gaining media attention.

• • •

If you want to learn more about the
Power over Pain program, you can visit their Website at:
www.painfoundation.org
and click on the Power over Pain link.

Detailed stories of advocacy can be found in the archives for the Pain Community News online newsletter at:

www.painfoundation.org/newletters/pain04fall.pdf

CHAPTER SIX

Lifting the Burden: A Global Campaign

Sarah had been learning about how individuals can help make the public more aware of the need for effective pain treatments. She came across programs that were being administered at both the state and national levels. Her eyes opened wide when she came across the next campaign. Now pain awareness campaigns have gone global. Lifting the Burden is a campaign aimed at the whole planet.

On March 26, 2004, after seven years of planning, the World Health Organization (WHO) in Copenhagen launched the global campaign called Lifting the Burden. This program was designed mainly for people with headache pain, which can be chronic in more serious cases. Some people suffer from constant headache pain that disrupts almost every part of their day-to-day lives. The benefits of this campaign have started to spread around the world and will help all people in pain.

Headache pain is a global problem. People from all over the world suffer from it. In recognition of this huge problem, the World Health Organization initiated talks with three other world organizations: The World Headache Alliance, the International Headache Society, and the European Headache Foundation. All these organizations joined together and committed themselves to fighting for better pain treatments across the globe.

Together these organizations set up this program, which is called Reducing the Burden of Headache Worldwide, or Lifting the Burden. This campaign involves seven basic steps. The first step is to acknowledge the huge scope of this problem. Dr. Timothy Steiner is the chairman of this global campaign. He wrote a review of this project in the prestigious scientific journal, Lancet Neurology, in 2004. In this article he discussed how headache pain is one of the top sources of disability throughout the world.

Some countries are more advanced in their treatment of headache pain than others, of course. Dr. Steiner pointed out, sadly, that in some places, headache disorders are not even recognized as a medical problem. One of the goals of this global campaign is to help reduce the large gaps that exist between the need for care and access to it.

Most of the steps in this campaign involve helping to educate the world about the many new treatment options that are becoming available to help sufferers of headache pain. This campaign is devoted to raising the information level worldwide about correct recognition and diagnosis of headache disorders. The campaign also educates the public in ways to avoid mismanagement of pain, in how to promote appropriate lifestyle modifications that can reduce the triggers for pain (e.g., migraines), and promotes the use of cost-effective treatments.

• • •

The Website for Lifting the Burden can be located by accessing the World Health Organization Website at:

www.who.int

At the homepage, type in the word "headache" in the Search box. You can also find detailed information pages about headaches from the link, WHO Fact Sheet No. 277 on headache disorders.

There is a link to the article by Dr. Timothy Steiner, originally published in Lancet Neurology. In this article Dr. Steiner, a neurologist, discusses the history and importance of this project. Further information can be found from the World Headache Alliance Website:

www.w-h-a.org

CHAPTER SEVEN

The Patient Pain Manifesto

On May 11, 2001, the Canadian Pain Society put out the following press release.

FOR IMMEDIATE RELEASE:

> Montreal, May 11, 2001: Within Canada's healthcare system, there exists a severe under-treatment of pain. To address this worrying situation, the Canadian Pain Society today launched an aggressive new initiative: The Patient Pain Manifesto. This public awareness and education campaign will be aimed at alerting and educating hospital patients and their families, regarding their rights in the management of their pain.

The press release from the Canadian Pain Society also described the intent of this program. "The Patient Pain Manifesto was developed by the Canadian Pain Society as a 'bill of rights' to clearly communicate to hospital patients and their families, their rights regarding treatment of pain resulting from surgery, treatment, or illness" (Johnston, 2001). This is a quote from Dr. Celeste Johnston, a professor at McGill University's School of Nursing in Montreal. At the time of this press release (2001), Dr. Johnston was also the president of the Canadian Pain

Society, an affiliate of the International Association for the Study of Pain. (This great organization will be described in detail later in Book Three.)

Dr. Johnston went on to say: "Studies show that a surprising number of patients believe that suffering is part of being in hospital and being ill. We want to make sure that patients with pain are fully aware that they have the right to receive treatment that will keep their pain under control, and help them reclaim their lives" (Johnston, 2001).

One of the central goals of this manifesto is to provide education, awareness, and advocacy about pain and its impact on people's lives. These goals apply to the treatment of pain, not only in Canada, but around the world. Accurate information is also provided to dispel common myths about pain.

Some of the most common myths are:

- Pain is an accepted part of being in hospital.
- No pain, no gain; pain is part of healing.
- Patients will become addicted to painkillers.

Facts should be replacing these fictions.

The facts are that pain itself can be extremely harmful. It can result in more medical complications, longer hospital stays, greater disability, and potentially long-term pain. Persistent pain can be difficult to treat, but every attempt should be made to do so. It is easier to treat the pain when it is still in the early stages. Individuals should be given every option for pain relief to help avoid future complications and help avoid the potential for long-term pain.

The goals for this Canadian education and awareness campaign are to:

- Improve education of medical and nursing students during their training
- Provide more continuing education opportunities for healthcare professionals on the assessment and management of pain
- Work more closely with patients to determine their needs
- Work more closely with industry to help market educational materials
- Distribute a million book marks about this pain patient manifesto to patients, their families, and health professionals
- Distribute ten thousand posters to healthcare professionals and clinics. (Canadian Pain Society)

• • •

The Patient Pain Manifesto can be found at the Website for the Canadian Pain Society:
www.canadianpainsociety.ca
(look for the link under "News ")

Pain Explained – Update

A news release, November 3, 2008, announced a new campaign called Painexplained.ca, Getting Answers For Pain.

"When you or someone you love is suffering, every minute spent waiting for proper pain care feels like a travesty," said Lynn Cooper, President of the Canadian Pain Coalition and campaign founding member.

"We know that too many are not getting the timely care they desperately want and deserve," said Dr. Barry Sessle, President of the Canadian Pain Society and campaign co-founder.

Please check out this new Website. Painexplained.ca is a new campaign supported by the Canadian Pain Society, Canadian Pain Coalition, the Canadian Pain Foundation and other partners groups, companies and individuals. The campaign seeks to raise awareness and promote better prevention and management of all types of pain in Canada.

Of course, this information is available through the internet to everyone worldwide.

CHAPTER EIGHT

Pain: The Fifth Vital Sign

On November 11, 1995, Dr. James Campbell gave a presidential address to the American Pain Society in Los Angeles, California. In that address, he launched a new campaign to help promote more effective treatments for pain. He wanted to change not only the way medicine is practiced, but also the way doctors and nurses are trained.

All doctors and nurses know the importance of the four vital signs. These are temperature, respiration, pulse, and blood pressure. These vital signs help the doctor monitor how a particular patient is doing, no matter what illness or injury they may experience. These vital signs are necessary to monitor, especially at times of emergency. These signs are well known to emergency room doctors, triage nurses, trauma specialists, and paramedics.

Dr. Campbell felt that pain needed to be taken seriously at any time of emergency and also as an ongoing process in the treatment of patients' illnesses and injuries. He summed up this idea clearly in the following quote:

"Vital signs are taken seriously. If pain were assessed with the same zeal as other vital signs are, it would have a much better chance of being treated properly. We need to train doctors and nurses to treat pain as a vital sign. Quality care means that pain is measured and treated." (Campbell, 1995)

Since 1995, this Fifth Vital Sign campaign has helped to elevate the awareness of pain treatment among healthcare professionals. The campaign has encouraged medical professionals to take their patients' complaints of pain more seriously. Dr. Campbell reminded doctors not to put patients in the position of having to ask for a favor when they want pain relief. It is clear that Dr. Campbell is a true humanitarian.

Sarah could see the practical changes Dr. Campbell had started. Real progress is being made. In many hospitals throughout the world, pain is now treated seriously, as a fifth vital sign. There is still a long way to go, especially for insurance companies, but at least the journey had begun.

• • •

For more information about the Fifth Vital Sign campaign, click on the link (Advocacy) at the Website for the American Pain Society:

www.ampainsoc.org

CHAPTER NINE

Women in Pain Recognition. Respect. Relief.

The Women in Pain Initiative has amazing ideas and energy. It has a simple mission: to ensure the ethical and equal treatment of all women in pain.

The Women in Pain Initiative also has a larger vision – a very just and necessary vision. The first part is straightforward and is a common one seen in many campaigns to help promote awareness of the needs for effective pain treatments. Members of the Women in Pain Initiative want to ensure that women of all backgrounds have their pain managed effectively and without bias.

The second part of the group's vision really struck home with Sarah. She had been battling not only the myths and biases experienced by people in pain, but additional biases that were targeted toward her as a woman and single mother in pain.

The second part of the vision for the Women in Pain Initiative reads as follows:

> "Through these collective actions, all women in pain will no longer be victimized by cultural myths and professional misconceptions, which most often result in the discounting and/or

> dismissal of their pain reports as being "all in their heads," "psychogenic," "hysterical," "hormonal," or otherwise "not real," and may lead to serious or life threatening medical consequences."

As Sarah was reading this from their Website, she could feel her breath quicken. Her own feelings and history had been put so clearly into words. She didn't realize that this was such a widespread problem. Now she felt really charged up. She kept reading more about their vision.

> "All women in pain will be guaranteed a standard of care comparable to their male counterparts and will be allowed to express their pain experience in a way that is true to their nature, without fear of being labeled "too emotional."

Ultimately, the Women in Pain Initiative will enable all women to maintain the quality of their lives and to be empowered with the knowledge and self-dignity to demand this basic human right.

To bring this vision to light, this group had a very detailed action plan, with three main components: public awareness, healthcare professional education, and legislative action. In each of these domains there are clear objectives, an advocacy plan, and a list of tactics and communications. The details of each of these action plans are outlined on the group's Website. A media kit is provided to help individuals and professionals promote these ideas to the media. Women are also encouraged to share their stories on the Website. This sharing is an important form of support and helps women like Sarah understand that they are not alone in this often all-consuming war.

• • •

Please check out the incredible Women in Pain Initiative link from the following Website:
www.forgrace.org

CHAPTER TEN

Never Again: A Dream For Grace

Sarah was excited already. Then she came across this Website called For Grace: The Dream of Never Again. This is a very beautiful and creative Website.

It provides a lot of very detailed information about pain, especially the pain caused by RSD (Reflex Sympathetic Dystrophy, which has a new name, Complex Regional Pain Syndrome, CRPS).

Even the opening video graphics on this Website are gorgeous. As you can see from its homepage logo, a lot of energy and creativity has gone into this Website. In Sarah's dreams, she would love for her group's Website to be so impressive.

For Grace is a non-profit organization passionately devoted to raising public awareness of RSD.

It is estimated that between 1.5 and 1.6 million Americans suffer from the devastating chronic pain disease, Reflex Sympathetic Dystrophy. Yet to date, RSD remains virtually unknown.

For Grace was inspired by the true-life story of its founder and spokesperson, Cynthia Toussaint. She is a former ballerina who suffered with RSD for over twenty years, after a ballet injury. Ms. Toussaint is a champion of people with RSD and has been active with public speaking, media presentations, interviews, and political advocacy for those who do not have a voice. Her twenty-four year partner and caregiver, John Garrett, also assumes a leadership role in this organization.

This passionate organization is named after Grace, a sister of Cynthia's mother. She did not know her Aunt Grace, since Grace died before Cynthia was born. Cynthia was told that Grace's passing came too early and with too much pain. "She was only twenty years old, a life of promise quieted long before its blossom." These are the words of Cynthia who thought of Grace as a pure and simple angel. John and Cynthia dreamed of having a little girl and naming her after Aunt Grace. For Grace is named for the child that John and Cynthia were never able to have. Their organization is also dedicated with hope to all the Graces that will be born to women with RSD, who can have children once they are diagnosed early, treated, and cured. This is their dream and the foundation for their actions and creative drives. (This history is available on the For Grace Website).

In addition to the beauty and creativity, the For Grace Website and media kits provide detailed fact sheets about RSD, stories of women with RSD, and lists of resources and professionals who specialize in this area.

• • •

Sarah couldn't wait to show this information to her friends in the Website group. The Website can be found at:

www.forgrace.org

CHAPTER ELEVEN

The Pain Care Coalition

Sarah became aware that several of the biggest pain organizations were trying to pressure governments to provide better research and care for people in pain. This helped her to feel that significant steps were being taken in the right direction.

In one of her research adventures, she came across The Pain Care Coalition. This coalition was organized in June of 1998 and involved members from the American Pain Society, The American Association for Pain Medicine, and the American Association for the Study of Headache. Together, their mission was to create a task force to work toward influencing government regulations, research funding, and access to treatment.

One goal of the Pain Care Coalition is to alert professionals and policy makers to what happens on a week-by-week basis in Washington, D.C. The Coalition publishes a weekly newsletter and email distribution to describe new political developments. Specifically, they outline details related to new initiatives and changes in health law, public policy, research funding, and federal regulations regarding patients' rights, Medicare financing, research financing, and patients' access to adequate pain treatments.

These organizations are focused upon improving treatment and research for individuals in pain, by assisting healthcare professionals, politicians, and lawmakers. Sarah liked the idea of all parts of society working together to deliver better treatment and care for people in pain.

Sarah found out about The Pain Care Coalition through the American Pain Society Website:

www.ampainsoc.org

She found the details under their Advocacy and Policy section. Some of the materials she was reading were beyond her knowledge. She found it comforting, though, to know that there were many important and influential organizations working to help people like her.

There is also a Canadian Pain Care Coalition which can be found at **www.painexplained.ca** (described in Chapter Seven). There is a lot of detailed help, here, for people in pain.

CHAPTER TWELVE

Partners for Understanding Pain

Sarah dug deeper into her research and discovered more and more groups trying to help people in pain. There were the more professional organizations, discussed earlier, such as The American Pain Society and several associations for pain professionals. Then Sarah came across an organization whose members were people like her: the American Chronic Pain Association.

As explained in the Website, Penny Cowan founded the American Chronic Pain Association (ACPA) in 1980. She is from Pittsburgh, Pennsylvania and spent many years struggling with chronic pain. Treatment in the Cleveland Pain Clinic helped her learn many new skills that she wanted to share with others in pain.

Penny Cowan's mission started when she placed a notice in her church bulletin. She soon found others who needed help with their pain, and they began meeting in their first ACPA support group. This group grew quickly and new groups formed. Cowan could not help out directly in every group, so she developed manuals and handouts for members to use as they established their own groups. Today, there are several hundred chronic pain groups growing throughout Canada and the United States.

The American Chronic Pain Association created an impressive Website to help people around the world. It contains updated stories about new pain discoveries, new treatment strategies, and new funding initiatives for pain research. Videos are available to watch through the Website. Interviews with Penny Cowan and other people with pain reveal what strategies were successful and which strategies have not worked for them.

The ACPA has links to practical articles, which describe strategies to improve coping with pain. One article outlines ten simple and useful steps. Another article explains the factors involved in deciding how and when a multidisciplinary pain program might be beneficial.

The ACPA also began an education campaign called Partners for Understanding Pain. Partners is actually a group of organizations that are working together to help improve the personal, economic, and social circumstances of people in pain. The goal is to work with all members of society, not just professionals. Partners include groups that focus on specific health conditions as well as groups that have wider goals such as improving the lives of people with all types of chronic and acute pain conditions.

Partners for Understanding Pain receives support from several pharmaceutical firms. These companies help to distribute public education and awareness materials to individuals, hospitals, and pharmacists. The Website for the American Chronic Pain Association has a link where materials sponsored by Partners for Understanding Pain are available for download.

The Partners campaign has developed a comprehensive educational book called *In the Face of Pain: Pain Management Advocacy Tool Kit.* This book is over two hundred pages and is available free from the Website listed below.

The more Sarah researched, the more convinced she became that she was on the right track with her own Website ideas. Other people had similar ideas, which was a good sign. Even professionals and drug companies want to help educate others and improve the lives of people in pain. There is a lot of work to be done. Sarah was glad to have the support of these organizations and to know they are all working toward the same goal – here at home and around the world.

• • •

The book, *In the Face of Pain: Pain Management Advocacy Tool Kit* and information about Partners for Understanding Pain can be found at the homepage for The American Chronic Pain Association:
www.theacpa.org

CHAPTER THIRTEEN

Pain Care Minutes: National Radio Programs

Sarah heard about this next example from one of the people in her Internet group. The American Pain Society has created sixty-second radio programs called the Sixty-Second Check-Up. These shows include brief interviews, broadcast every Thursday on the radio. The host is Christopher Michael, and he often includes interviews with top scientists in the pain research field.

The Sixty-Second Check-Up involves short interviews that are easy to understand and often entertaining. Recent interviews have covered topics such as:

- Treating Chronic Pain in Children, by Dr. Patricia McGrath
- Chronic Pain is America's Number One Health Problem, by Dr. Richard Payne
- Hospitals are Putting More Emphasis on Treating Pain, by Dr. Dennis Turk
- Who "Feels" More Pain than Our Women?, by Dr. Gerry Gebhart
- Racial Disparities In Pain Management, by Dr. Carmen Green
- Patient–Doctor Communication Influences Pain
- Management Success, by Dr. Judith Paice

Sarah was intrigued when she found out about these interviews, but disappointed because she thought that she had missed them. Of course, it is difficult to be available at a specific time to listen to the interviews being broadcast on the radio. Fortunately, the Website of The American Pain Society: **www.ampainsoc.org** has a listing of the recent interviews and are easily available to view from the Website using the Pain Care Minutes Radio Programs link. Free software to view the programs is also available through the Website.

Sarah was starting to feel that some real work has been done in this area. Finally, some very important messages are getting out to the people in need – in a very people-friendly way.

Pain Care Minutes can be accessed through the Website for the American Pain Society:

www.ampainsoc.org

CHAPTER FOURTEEN

Chronic Pain and the Law

When Sarah first found this Website, she felt a little beyond her depth. This seemed to be a heavy-duty site aimed mostly at legal scholars and professionals. As she kept reading, however, she found there were sections for people in pain, also for lawyers, doctors, and politicians.

This Website (based on United States law) was developed by The Center for Health Law Studies at St. Louis University, in combination with The American Society of Law, Medicine and Ethics. It is funded by a grant from the May-Day fund. There is a section on breaking news. This includes excerpts from different journals as well as archives for accessing previous postings and articles.

Some of these news articles relate to legal and ethical topics. For example, one article discussed various legal issues regarding the use of pain medications. Here, some doctors described feeling at risk for a lawsuit if they prescribed pain medications for their patients in need. Other doctors felt more at risk for under-prescribing. This is a difficult dilemma for doctors and one that directly affects individuals in pain. This article, called "Why is Our Government Pursuing a War on Doctors?" was posted by David Brushwood.

Under the section entitled, *For Persons in Pain*, there is more practical and day-to-day information, and links to other sites where individuals can find some much needed help. The legal and ethical areas may be beyond the understanding of many people, yet it is still comforting to know that these issues are being discussed and that these advocacy campaigns exist. Sarah wanted to make sure that no area of publicity and education was left out.

• • •

The Pain and the Law Website can be found at:
www.painandthelaw.org

Canadians may want to read an excellent book by Dr. Mary Lynch, *Surviving your personal injuries, claim and litigation: A Guide Book* (2003).

CHAPTER FIFTEEN

My Pain: A Project from the National Pain Foundation

Sarah found that this Website was one of the most useful of all. There was even a heading in the first paragraph of the "My Pain" link:

If You Are In Crisis, Click Here.

This Website has a wealth of accurate and up-to-date information that individuals can use for themselves or take to their healthcare provider. This kind of detailed information helps individuals take a more active role in their pain treatment. The basic philosophy is the more you know about your pain condition, the better prepared you will be to manage your pain. Individuals can even sign up to receive a free monthly email newsletter.

At the top of the Website homepage, individuals are encouraged to select a pain category where they can learn more up-to-date information. There is a listing of several categories of pain where individuals can find out more about their specific injuries and illnesses. There are links that outline different treatment options, tips for finding a pain specialist, and details on how to create and record a personal pain journal. There is also a link called the "Personal Pain Inventory." This is an interactive survey that helps individuals to record all the details of their particular injury, the history of their pain, the details of where and when it hurts, and the types of treatments they have tried. This can be an ongoing and permanent record for individuals to show to their healthcare provider or even their lawyer.

• • •

This information and much more, is available from a main link on the National Pain Foundation Website:

www.nationalpainfoundation.org

This comprehensive Website was described in more detail in chapter three.

CHAPTER SIXTEEN

Your Own Pain Information Library

This link has been created and sponsored by the American Pain Foundation. The Pain Information Library link has detailed information about various types of pain and the illnesses that cause pain. The library has up-to-date articles about finding appropriate care, medications, the impact of pain on women in society, and discussions and information about complementary and alternative medicines.

The American Pain Foundation made this link available as part of its mission to eliminate the under-treatment of pain in America. The foundation also offers a free newsletter that can be sent by mail or by email, called *Pain Community News.* (This was described in chapter four.) This newsletter has a great deal of detailed information about education campaigns, injuries, illnesses, and about all the activities organized throughout America. Since pain is a worldwide problem, this information is useful to all people in pain, no matter where they live.

Through the Website you can also watch a video called *Voices of People with Pain.* This is easy to do by clicking on the link from their Website. If you need some extra software to watch this video on your computer, the software can be easily downloaded, free of charge, with the link that is provided. Sarah thought that having a video available was a great idea. A video makes the stories and experiences more real. It really helps people who feel alone in their struggle with pain and injury.

• • •

Links to the Pain Information Library, *Voices of the People,* and the free newsletter can be found on the Website of the American Pain Foundation at:

www.painfoundation.org

CHAPTER SEVENTEEN

Brainstorm

Brainstorm is a multimedia educational program. It is based on specific patient cases and uses illustrations from case studies and animation to show the impact of headaches on patients' lives. This program is very specific in scope. First of all, it is focused on educating physicians and healthcare professionals. Secondly, it is focused mostly on pain related to headaches. This is understandable, since the program has been set up and is managed by the American Headache Society.

The Brainstorm program includes up-to-date information on the diagnosis and treatment of patients with complex migraine disorders. The medical information in this program is designed mainly for professionals to learn all the new information necessary to provide the best kind of treatment for patients suffering from various types of headaches. Since this information is available on the Internet, it can help physicians and their patients around the globe.

Brainstorm provides an excellent example of how the Internet is used to assist in providing physicians and healthcare professionals all the up-to-date information needed to administer the highest quality of pain treatment. Most of the well-known pain societies and organizations around the world also provide detailed information to professionals.

Another good example comes from The American Pain Society. The society has created a public policy statement on the rights and responsibilities of healthcare professionals in the use of opioid medication for the treatment of pain. This is a highly controversial area. The American Pain Society has joined together with The American Academy of Pain Medicine and The American Society of Addiction Medicine to provide some guidelines for physicians who feel uncertain and vulnerable when they are prescribing strong pain medications to help their patients. There is detailed medical information presented in these education programs, as well as a support network for professionals who want to ensure they are doing everything possible to help their patients in the safest way.

Yet another example can be found on the Website from The American Academy of Pain Medicine. This campaign is called The Physician's Voice in Pain Medicine. It represents a medical society for physicians practicing in the field of pain medicine and helps with education, training, advocacy, and research. The goal of this organization and its education campaigns is to help physicians from a variety of specialties who have a common interest in pain medicine. These medical specialties include anesthesiology, internal medicine, neurology, neurological surgery, orthopaedic surgery, physiatry, and psychiatry. Other professions can benefit as well, of course.

Much of this medical information was too complex for Sarah to grasp. She was glad she came across this Website, however. It helped to boost her confidence and hope that doctors and scientists cared about people in pain, and to know that doctors from around the world were working together to find better treatments.

• • •

Information about The Physician's Voice in Pain Medicine can be found at:

www.painmed.org

The Brainstorm program is outlined on the Website for the American Headache Society at:

www.ahsnet.org/brainstorm.php

CHAPTER EIGHTEEN

Pain Relief Is a Human Right

Dr. Frank Brennan and Dr. Michael Cousins wrote an article called: "Pain Relief Is a Human Right." It was written for a newsletter from The International Association for the Study of Pain, called *Pain: Clinical Updates*, appearing in September 2004.

Sarah shuddered when she came across this article. She liked the authors' emphasis on the need for more effective treatments, of course. Yet it was the bigger message that really hit home for Sarah. She learned about a worldwide movement organized to fight against the under-treatment of pain. The goal was to ensure that pain relief is understood as a universal right.

The two big movers have been the International Association for the Study of Pain and the World Health Organization. Drs. Brennan and Cousins state:

> "The time has come. The problem is clear. Pain is a major public health issue throughout the world. The gap between an increasingly sophisticated knowledge of pain and its treatment and the effective application of that knowledge is large and widening." (Brennan & Cousins, 2004)

We are learning more and more about pain and how to treat it. Unfortunately, there is an ever-increasing gap between what we know and can provide, and what is actually provided for people in pain.

This war is fought on several fronts. As we have seen throughout the earlier chapters, there has been a large push toward a greater education about the types of pain that need treatments and the new treatments that are being discovered each day. There is also a pressure for medical students to learn more about pain early on in their medical education. It is not enough for them to learn about pain in their specialty training. Even early medical education, and the training of family physicians, needs to have a clear emphasis on the treatment and management of pain.

There is pressure being placed on governments and hospital administrations for patients to receive effective pain management. It is no longer enough to have the cause of their pain treated. It is necessary to have the pain itself treated. This is especially important for long-term (or chronic) pain, where the cause of the individual's pain cannot be cured.

This battle is also fought on the international level. Professional healthcare and regulatory societies throughout the world are working together and promoting universal pain management standards. Government action and reform is on its way to make it easier for doctors to prescribe pain medications when necessary. There is also pressure to reduce the costs of pain medications.

For now, it is important to enforce the rights that have already been recognized in national and international laws. Policies from the United Nations, as an example, have made it clear in their Universal Declaration of Human Rights (1948). Similar policies have appeared in the International Covenant on Civil and Political Rights (1966) and the International Covenant on Economic Social and Cultural Rights (1966). The covenant explains the right "of everyone to the enjoyment of the highest attainable standard of physical and mental health." The overall goal is to ensure that as a society we use all the methods available to provide for the relief of pain and the promotion of health. (These documents are reviewed in Brennan and Cousins, 2004).

This movement felt right to Sarah. There is still a large battle to be fought when it comes to discovering new and more effective methods for the relief of pain. We should not have to fight for the treatment methods that have already been discovered. There is a great deal to be learned and a great deal to be done.

Sarah was glad to know that she is not alone in trying to help the millions of people in pain. As she came across Websites and articles, pain organization after organization, she realized that much is already being done all around the world. It helped Sarah to know that she was a part of this inspiring movement. She couldn't wait to share all these amazing discoveries with Suzanne, Ashley, and Mike.

Part Two:

Learning from Doctors in Pain

CHAPTER ONE

Dr. Devin Starlanyl and Mary Ellen Copeland

Much can be learned from the research conducted by doctors and scientists. New ideas and treatments are discovered by scientific research every day. Doctors who live in pain can also provide special insights. Dr. Devin Starlanyl is one of these doctors who has had the courage to come forward and describe, not only her personal experience and knowledge about chronic pain, but also her understanding of the medical research that has been rapidly progressing in this field.

Dr. Starlanyl's first book about fibromyalgia, *Fibromyalgia and Chronic Myofascial Pain: A Survival Manual,* was a huge success. She wrote this book in 1996 with Mary Ellen Copeland. Both of these authors live with daily pain and limitations caused by fibromyalgia, and are also experts in their field – an unbeatable combination.

Dr. Starlanyl did her formal medical training in emergency room medicine. She has also done hospice and public health work. Her struggles with pain have brought about serious limitations in her life. She has not been able to practice full-time medicine since 1993. She is only able to work on writing and consulting projects, on a very part-time basis. Personal experience has taught her about the difficult struggles with pain and illness, as well as how debilitating fibromyalgia and chronic myofascial pain can be. (Both of these medical conditions cause multiple chronic pain symptoms and related limitations.) It is the combination of her medical background and her personal experiences that have allowed her to bring a very sound understanding and compassionate approach to her writings about pain.

Mary Ellen Copeland also brings personal experience and expert knowledge to her writings about fibromyalgia. She lives with this condition on a daily basis and has had much of her life disrupted by pain. She is a distinguished teacher, writer, and lecturer and has also written several books about depression. She made a video entitled *Cope with Depression*, which is widely used by therapists.

The first book written by Devin Starlanyl and Mary Ellen Copeland is an amazing book. It is not hard to understand why it has become so popular. It is indeed a comprehensive survival manual. This book describes the medical facts and patterns associated with fibromyalgia and myofascial pain syndrome, the symptoms, and why they occur. Although written for patients, it provides a wealth of information to assist doctors and therapists with accurate identification and diagnosis of these types of chronic pain. As these authors point out, "The average FMS (fibromyalgia syndrome) patient suffers for five years and spends thousands of dollars on medical bills before receiving an accurate diagnosis. As a result of misdiagnosis, more than half of all patients undergo unnecessary surgery" (Starlanyl & Copeland, 1996, 2001).

Long-term pain is the primary symptom of fibromyalgia, but not the only one. These authors explain how this type of chronic pain can affect sleep and many other bodily functions. They also help readers to understand the role of stress and describe many different healing tools. Such tools include descriptions and discussions about relaxation, meditation, nutrition, and other helpful alternatives. Importantly, the authors also discuss the necessity of advocacy, both for patients themselves and on behalf of the many people in the patients' lives who are affected.

In a second book written by Dr. Starlanyl, she takes this advocacy a leap further. In 1999, she published *The Fibromyalgia Advocate.* This book includes even stronger recommendations and detailed information about how individuals can advocate for themselves and fight for their rights.

When Sarah discovered this book, she felt an instant connection. She knew Ashley would, too. They both knew how hard it was to fight for their rights with doctors and insurance companies. In her book, Dr. Starlanyl describes the rights that people have with regard to disability benefits, healthcare treatments, and support in the workplace. Not surprisingly, this book has also been a tremendous success. It adds credibility for all victims of chronic pain; individuals who are struggling to get a fair shake with their insurance companies and their workplace. It is clear from these writings that Dr. Starlanyl has a solid base of knowledge and a deep core of compassion. From her personal experiences with pain, her medical background, and her comprehensive books, she has been able to help many people fight for what is just and fair. Thousands of people have benefited from having such a talented and caring fighter as their advocate.

• • •

These books are available through libraries, many bookstores or for purchase through the following Website:

www.sover.net/~devstar/

Dr. Starlanyl has also just finished writing the chapter on Chronic Myofascial Pain for the upcoming third edition of Travell and Simon's Myofascial Pain and Dysfunction. She has studied pain caused by myofascial trigger points, extensively, and describes how treatments targeted toward trigger points can provide significant relief for some patients.

Lets all hope that Dr. Devin Starlanyl and Mary Ellen Copeland have the strength to keep writing. They truly help make the world a better place.

CHAPTER TWO

Dr. Mark J. Pellegrino

Dr. Pellegrino is a fibromyalgia survivor and a fighter – for his own life, and for the health of his patients. He has struggled to cope with this painful illness for many years and understands how long-term pain can seep into every corner of life.

He has advanced medical training, is a specialist in physical medicine and rehabilitation, and spends his working days helping people cope with pain and disability. He has diagnosed and treated thousands of patients with fibromyalgia and other painful conditions.

Dr. Pellegrino has written several books on fibromyalgia. They are all easy to understand and spell out the symptoms, limitations, and treatment options for fibromyalgia. One of his more recent books, *Understanding Post-traumatic Fibromyalgia*, caught Sarah's eye as she was "surfing the Web." She found a reference to this book and felt that it would be perfect for Ashley. In it, Dr. Pellegrino outlines different types of fibromyalgia and identifies a specific type as being post-traumatic in nature. He describes post-traumatic fibromyalgia as a special category of fibromyalgia, commonly seen following a trauma such as a motor vehicle accident or a work injury. Sarah knew Ashley had developed fibromyalgia after her motor vehicle accident and couldn't wait to share this news about Dr. Pellegrino and his books with her.

This doctor is also a compassionate advocate for people who suffer from chronic pain and fibromyalgia. He knows the scientific literature and challenges any medical expert who claims that fibromyalgia does not exist.

> "If a physician tries to state an "expert opinion" that fibromyalgia does not exist, he or she will not be in compliance with the current scientific standard of knowledge. A knowledgeable attorney can portray this doctor's testimony as unreliable and not consistent with factual scientific knowledge." (Pellegrino, 1996)

Dr. Pellegrino knows the truth about this type of chronic pain from his medical knowledge, the scientific research, and from his own experiences living every day with pain. This deep knowledge base allows his books to be both supportive and informed. It is obvious he believes patients should receive fair treatment and disability benefits when they cannot work.

He is very clear in his books that fibromyalgia is a real, physical, and medical condition and describes how stress is not considered to be a cause. Yet, once an individual does have fibromyalgia or other types of chronic pain, their lives can be filled up with stress. These are secondary stresses that come after an individual has been suffering from pain, limitations, and often many losses. These stresses occur after the onset of the illness and are not the cause. Dr. Pellegrino emphasizes this important point in all his writings.

For Sarah, Ashley, Mike, and Suzanne, this point was emphasized during the hospital pain program. Stress is a common source of aggravation for most of the physical injuries and illnesses that cause pain. It can also weaken a person by interfering with their sleep, energy, memory, and ability to cope. But stress is not the cause of fibromyalgia, as Dr. Pellegrino explains, nor is it the cause of any type of chronic pain. Sarah was glad to read that he was clear about this issue. It felt good to know that the experts were on her side.

• • •

Dr. Pellegrino's books about fibromyalgia include:
Understanding Post-traumatic Fibromyalgia
Fibromyalgia: Up Close and Personal
The Fibromyalgia Survivor
Laugh at your Muscles I and II
A Sunnier Tomorrow

These books are all published by Anadem Publications and can be found through the Website:

www.anadem.com/fibro.html

Sarah was able to find some of these books in the library and a friend also had the *Fibromyalgia Survivor.* Often these books can be bought used through Amazon (www.amazon.com). Sarah knew that these books could be a big help for Ashley.

CHAPTER THREE

Kristin Thorson and the Fibromyalgia Network

The first thing Sarah noticed when she opened the homepage for the Fibromyalgia Network Website was this:

> Fibromyalgia Network takes your pain,
> fatigue, and brain-fog symptoms seriously!

Wow, thought Sarah. The writers of this Website know how hard it is to not be taken seriously. This is one of the strong fears that many individuals with chronic pain and fibromyalgia experience. Their symptoms and limitations are always challenged. This issue is so important that the writers of this Website felt it was necessary to put this message front and center.

Further down the homepage, two other items jumped out at Sarah and made the same central point.

> Your fibromyalgia symptoms are real. Learn
> how patients handle credibility issues.

> Research tests can validate your symptoms
> and possible causes.

These messages are highlighted to provide validation and support for individuals suffering from fibromyalgia. Part of each message includes a link to three free articles on fibromyalgia, all related to the reality of this condition.

It is clear from the Website's homepage that the Fibromyalgia Network is not a free service. Aside from offering real and important help for people, this network is a business selling a newsletter and a membership. To be fair, this is a very reasonable offer. With a one-year membership, individuals receive a free newsletter plus other free services, all at a cost of twenty-eight dollars per year.

Although this is a business, Sarah was glad to see that the newsletter did not contain any advertisements or other promotions. In fact, the Fibromyalgia Network is very strict about this issue. Those wanting to advertise in the newsletter, or to purchase subscriber mailing lists to sell products to subscribers, approach the group on a regular basis. The response to all requests is always a stern no. This is an important protective mechanism to ensure members and readers are not exposed to products that provide false claims or trivialize how people in pain feel. The mission here is clear. "We aim to educate and assist patients with ad-free, patient-focused information that they can put to use today." (Fibromyalgia Network) An important part of the network's mission is to protect members against exposure to harmful information from individuals wanting to sell products.

The Fibromyalgia Network has been a driving force in educating the world about fibromyalgia. It has been twenty years since this network and newsletter were created. To celebrate this milestone, the Fibromyalgia Network did a large survey of its members. Over thirty-five hundred members completed this survey with very encouraging results.

"Hope is gaining momentum." Treatments have improved. There is a greater awareness and understanding of fibromyalgia. People with fibromyalgia are supported more by their families and friends. "Doctors are starting to believe me, treat me better as a person, and work with me as a patient." This is just some of the good news drawn from this large survey, and reported in the April 2008 issue of the Fibromyaliga Network journal:

www.fmnetwork.com

A Little Background

As outlined on their Website, the Fibromyalgia Network started out as a newsletter created by Kristin Thorson. The first newsletter was created in 1988. This was a volunteer effort by Thorson, who went to meetings to learn about fibromyalgia and included this information in her newsletter.

This work was also very personal for her. She was diagnosed with fibromyalgia in 1986, at the young age of twenty-nine. Like the other doctors and writers described in earlier chapters, she knows from direct experience, what she is writing about. It was especially hard to be fighting this illness back in the 1980s. With her dedication, though, significant improvements have been made over the past twenty years. Now, more than ever, fibromyalgia is recognized as a real physical disorder.

Kristin Thorson is still the editor and an active contributor to articles in popular magazines to help educate the public about fibromyalgia. In 1991, the

Fibromyalgia Network began hosting information booths at major medical conferences to provide an important service – to help educate both the individuals who suffer from fibromyalgia and the medical and healthcare communities. These information booths often show up at conferences for rheumatologists, physiatrists, and family physicians. These volunteer efforts help educate and spread the news on updated research findings and sources.

As Sarah learned in her research on chronic pain, there are still many myths and misunderstandings prevalent for all types of conditions related to long-term pain. Fibromyalgia seems to attract more than its fair share of these myths. Formal diagnostic criteria for fibromyalgia were published in 1990 by the American Rheumatology Association. Scientists and doctors are still trying to understand the physical mechanisms responsible for this syndrome. Like other types of chronic pain, there is still much to learn. In the face of such uncertainties, there are many individuals, both in the medical community and in society at large, who have trouble understanding and accepting that such a condition can exist and affect millions of people.

The founders of the Fibromyalgia Network realized there were further obstacles at work. The major funding agency for scientific health research in the United States, the National Institutes of Health, had refused for many years to fund any research studies on fibromyalgia. This meant almost no research could take place, since many investigators did not have any private charity or related sources of funding to pay for their projects.

In 1993, the Fibromyalgia Network set out to launch a nationwide campaign to lobby both the United States House of Representatives and the Senate. This was an ambitious effort that continued for several years. Finally, some good news was reported on the Fibromyalgia Network Website. "After five years of working with patients across the country to lobby congress, the National Institutes of Health finally began to award several million dollars per year in research grants." (Fibromyalgia Network) Clearly the Fibromyalgia Network has gone many steps beyond basic education and has created an impact on the United States government and the major funding agencies, opening the door to research funding for fibromyalgia, which will benefit millions of patients and provide resources to healthcare providers.

• • •

More information about this impressive network and its membership benefits is available at:
www.fmnetwork.com

More information about Kristen Thorson's work with the Fibromyalgia Network can be found in her article, *I offered to write a newsletter*, Fibromyalgia Network Journal, October 2008.

Part Three:

Learning from Scientists

CHAPTER ONE

The Largest Investigation Ever Done

Sarah found a gold mine.

She couldn't wait to tell Mike. He had had his share of encounters with workers' compensation over the years. After his treatments with Evelyn, though, his ideas and relationship with workers' compensation improved considerably. Sarah was glad to be able to give him some of the news she had found. Mike was thrilled when he learned that the Workplace Safety and Insurance Board in Ontario, Canada had actually conducted the largest scientific study of chronic pain.

The research Sarah unearthed was huge. In three volumes, this study summarized all that was known about chronic pain at the time. This research was done by a panel of scientific experts put together through the Institute for Work and Health, which is part of the Workplace Safety and Insurance Board. Scientists from the institute reviewed more than eleven thousand five hundred articles from the scientific literature on chronic pain, which were all fairly recent and written between 1966 and August 1998. Then, the institute's scientists took these articles and abstracts and reduced them down to four hundred twelve high-quality research studies and endeavored to ensure each was based on clear scientific evidence. Sarah was amazed at how thorough and comprehensive these scientists had been in reviewing this pain research. She was also shocked to find out just how many studies were done on chronic pain, in hospitals and universities from around the world.

Findings from the Chronic Pain Initiative were reported in three volumes.

Report of the Chair of the Chronic Pain Panels (August 2000)

This is a summary of the research, findings, and recommendations from the Chronic Pain Initiative. It was prepared by the Chair of the Chronic Pain Panels, Brock Smith.

Report of the Chronic Pain Expert Advisory Panel (February 2000)

This book includes the scientific details, findings, and recommendations from the scientists who did this study. It includes definitions of chronic pain, causes and long-term outcomes of chronic pain, and sections on treatment, prevention, and disability management. Different scientific experts in the field wrote the chapters. The findings are clearly documented, and there are references to corroborate each of the findings from the scientific literature.

Report of the Chronic Pain Policy Advisory Panel (February 2000)

The third volume from the Chronic Pain Initiative involves recommendations for the future. Advisors with the Workplace Safety and Insurance Board wanted to use this research information to improve the ways in which the board helped injured workers.

This was a lot of reading for Sarah to go through, understandably. Of course, she was most interested in the scientific findings from the expert advisory panel. She wanted to use some of this information to put on her Website to help people who suffer from chronic pain. In her own struggles to cope with pain, she found it helped to know there were many scientists around the world working hard to find a cure for her injuries. It was also important to know progress was being made. Hope was hard to come by, especially at times when her pain symptoms were severely flared up. Hope was a necessary ingredient for her recovery and rehabilitation; it gave her that boost of energy she needed to keep moving forward.

With help from other members of her Website group, she tried to read through these three large volumes of research findings. Some of the highlights are included below.

Highlights from the Chronic Pain Experts Report

Definition of Chronic Pain

Chronic pain is defined as pain that persists six months after an injury and beyond the usual recovery time of a comparable injury; this pain may continue in the presence or absence of demonstrable pathology.

The main idea here is that doctors and scientists cannot always find objective evidence for the specific injury or illness that is causing a person's pain. Even when physical evidence of injury or illness cannot be found, it is still reasonable to consider the pain as being chronic, if it lasts longer than six months. Sometimes, even sophisticated MRIs cannot detect the source of a person's pain.

How Many People Are Affected?

The evidence suggests that as many as seventeen percent of the population suffer from chronic pain. This is a general estimate. Some types of pain are more common than others, of course. Back and neck pains are some of the more common types.

New Spinal Pain Research

In the past few years, there have been amazing advances toward the understanding of chronic pain disorders. In Australia, some studies have described new diagnostic techniques that have helped to identify a specific diagnosis in approximately sixty percent of patients with low back pain. These diagnostic techniques are quite new and require special training and facilities to administer.

In another series of Australian studies, new diagnostic techniques were able to identify approximately fifty percent of specific injuries that had caused chronic neck pain following whiplash injuries. Some early studies have also used spinal injections to treat chronic neck pain. These studies are still experimental at this stage, but show that some new and exciting work has been done.

Dr. Robert Teasell provides an excellent summary of new research findings to explain some of the possible physical causes for chronic neck and back pain, and fibromyalgia. His chapter in the *Chronic Pain Expert*

Report is entitled "Pathophysiology of Chronic Pain Disorders." The amount of detailed biological and neurological research that was done all over the world in these areas is truly exciting.

Chronic Pain is More than Just Pain

Dr. Warren Nielson wrote an excellent chapter entitled "The Concept of Pain." He outlines the long history of theories, which have tried to explain the causes and nature of chronic pain. Many of the early theories date back as far as Aristotle (384–322 BC), including the theories of Descartes (1664), which were often purely physical theories. They were mostly centered on pain itself and did not go very far in explaining chronic pain, its complexity, or how it differs from short-term pain.

As Dr. Nielson explains, short- and long-term pains have many differences. The obvious difference relates to how long the pain lasts. Chronic pain is typically defined as pain that lasts more than six months. It becomes more complicated as time goes on. Often, there are more stresses and losses as pain symptoms and related limitations continue to interfere with a person's life. These stresses keep building and serve to aggravate the individual's painful injuries or illness.

As these stresses build, there is a continuation and often a repeated aggravation of the individual's pain symptoms. Then, additional problems can arise, such as depression, loss of employment, financial stress, and family disruption. To understand the true nature of chronic pain, one needs to look at the whole picture. By only looking at the physical component, even though the physical injury or illness may be the original cause, doctors are not able to see clearly just how debilitating the chronic pain injury has become. Over time, injured individuals suffer not only from the original pain symptoms, but also from the secondary stresses and widespread interference with many aspects of their day-to-day lives.

Psychological Factors?

The workers' compensation system has been interested in the possibility that chronic pain can be caused by psychological factors and not necessarily by physical work injuries. If this were true, the workers' compensation system could save itself hundreds of millions of dollars by not paying for any compensation or benefits to individuals who suffer from chronic pain.

Dr. Klaus Kuch reviewed the many research studies that have investigated this possibility. He reviews these studies and describes the findings in a chapter entitled "Psychological Factors in Chronic Pain and Chronic Pain Disability." Below are some of his conclusions:

- There is inadequate evidence to support the theory that chronic pain results from prior psychiatric disorder.
- There is no scientific evidence that chronic depression is responsible for the development of low back pain, abdominal pain, or temporomandibular joint disorder. There was some evidence found that depression may be a predictor for the development of headache and chest pain, but this evidence was very limited and there were some weaknesses in the research that was conducted.

These weaknesses limited any possible conclusions regarding the effects of depression on the development of pain.

- Childhood abuse has long been suspected as a potential predictor of later health problems, including psychiatric disorder and pain. There is no scientific evidence to show that childhood sexual abuse is a cause of chronic pain.
- Several scientific studies were done to investigate whether additional stresses after a motor vehicle accident made it more difficult for individuals to recover from pain and disability. The evidence did show that extra stresses and distress did make it more difficult for individuals with pain to recover.
- There is evidence that when individuals in pain develop further problems related to depression, anxiety, and feelings of loss of control, that these additional stresses may slow their recovery from pain and their return to work. (Kuch, 2000)

These findings are not surprising. It is hard enough for individuals to cope with chronic pain itself, let alone having to cope with pain plus additional stressful events. These findings also match the experiences of Suzanne, Mike, Sarah, and Ashley described earlier in this book.

Overall, Dr. Kuch concludes:

"Psychological impairment may precede injury. It may also be a part of emerging chronic pain. Its presence does not prove that it has a role as a causative agent for chronic pain, although it clearly makes matters worse.

Poor psychological health can be a complication of pain that becomes apparent at an early stage of chronic pain." (Kuch, 2000)

Essentially, he is saying that, even if a person has had psychological or psychiatric problems in the past, there is no scientific evidence to show that these problems cause chronic pain.

The report of the Chronic Pain Experts Advisory Panel is a huge document. In addition to the chapters on research related to the causes of chronic pain, there are also chapters related to treatment, prevention, and the reduction of disability associated with various types of chronic pain. There are recommendations made to the Workplace Safety and Insurance Board and an extensive list of references documenting the scientific studies reviewed and used in this report.

Overall, it is very encouraging to see such great work being done. When scientists, doctors, and policy makers base their policies on solid scientific findings, there is a better chance that all injured workers will receive fair benefits and the best treatments available. This large investigation will help all individuals in pain. It is an amazing body of work.

CHAPTER TWO

The World's Top Pain Researchers

Sarah always enjoyed listening to David Letterman and his Top Ten List. She never would have dreamed, however, that someone would have created a list of the top ten pain researchers in the world. Yet, this was exactly what she found one day as she was organizing all the papers and articles she had gathered for her Website.

Three researchers from the psychology department at the University of Regina in Saskatchewan, Canada, of all places, put together this Top Ten List. They are Dr. Gordon Asmundson, Dr. Thomas Hadjistavropoulos, and Miranda Antonishyn. Their research and subsequent article appeared in the journal, *The Pain Clinic* in 2001.

To create this Top Ten List, these researchers used a very organized and scientific approach. They sent out a survey to members of the International Association for the Study of Pain and asked members to nominate individuals, whom they considered to be the current leading contributors in the field of pain. These questionnaires were sent to pain scientists from all over the world.

When all the data from the questionnaires were organized and put together, a list of the top ten individuals was created. Two individuals chose to not have their names listed in *The Pain Clinic* article. Their privacy was respected and only the top cight scientists were profiled.

Below is a list of each of these scientists in alphabetical order and a brief summary of their contributions. This information, taken from the article by Drs. Asmundson and Hadjistavropoulos, and Ms. Antonishyn, was published in *The Pain Clinic* article.

Allan Basbaum, Ph.D.

Dr. Basbaum was born in Montreal, Québec and attended McGill University. His first work in the field of pain research was under the guidance of Dr. Ronald Melzack. Dr. Basbaum went on to complete his doctorate at the University of Pennsylvania and subsequently worked with top scientists Dr. Patrick Wall and Dr. Howard Fields. Dr. Basbaum is currently Professor and Chair of the Department of Anatomy at the University of California in San Francisco.

He specializes in the study of pain and investigates the anatomical and neurological mechanisms responsible for how pain signals are transmitted. He has focused his studies on how persistent pain states develop and operate on a molecular level. The long-term goal of his research is to help develop treatments for individuals who suffer from different types of long-term clinical pain conditions.

John D. Loeser, MD

Dr. Loeser was born in Newark, New Jersey. He graduated from Harvard University and went on to complete medical training at New York University Medical School. He currently has a faculty position at the

University of Washington and is Professor of Neurological Surgery and Anesthesia. He has served as presidents of the International Association for the Study of Pain in the mid-1990s and was president of the American Pain Society in the mid-1980s. He is currently on the editorial board for several journals including *Pain, Neurosurgery,* and the *Journal of Musculoskeletal Pain.*

Dr. Loeser has conducted high-level research, both at a basic level in neuro-pharmacology and neurophysiology. Some of this research focuses on spinal cord nerve damage. He has also been active in studying chronic pain and working in a multidisciplinary pain center. He is a rare individual who can do basic research investigations and develop new clinical and treatment choices for people in pain.

Ronald Melzack, Ph.D.

Dr. Melzack was born in Montreal, Québec. He completed his undergraduate and graduate training in experimental psychology under the guidance of Dr. Donald Hebb at McGill University in Montreal. Early in his career, he also collaborated with Dr. Patrick Wall. He is now Professor Emeritus and Research Director of the Montreal General Hospital Pain Centre, plus was co-founder of the Royal Victoria Hospital's Pain Clinic.

Dr. Melzack has won numerous prestigious honors and awards. He has a special interest in investigating pain mechanisms in humans and investigating the role of the sympathetic nerve system in chronic and acute pain. Dr. Melzack has done research investigating pain mechanisms related to labor pain and phantom limb pain. He is well known for his groundbreaking research with Dr. Patrick Wall in the development of the gate control theory of pain and later on for his theory of the neuromatrix. The gate control theory set the stage for a revolution, both in the study and the treatment of pain.

Dr. Melzack has dedicated himself to the understanding of pain for almost half a century. In April 2009, he was inducted into the Canadian Medical Hall of Fame. The following quote was from the induction ceremony: "In 1965, he developed a new theory of pain (the gate control theory) that led to an explosion of pain research." In a recent interview, Dr. David Dozois paid tribute to Dr. Melzack: "It is his empathy for those suffering from chronic pain however that is perhaps his greatest gift of all" (Dozois, 2009). Interestingly, Dr. Melzack has also written three children's books retelling Eskimo legends, one of which has been made into a feature animated film.

Harold Merskey, DM

Dr. Merskey was born in Sunderland, England and received several undergraduate and graduate degrees, including his Doctor of Medicine, all from Oxford University. During his early career, he served as psychiatrist and consultant at two psychiatric institutions in England, followed by a long appointment at the National Hospital for Neurology and Neurosurgery. Currently, he is Professor Emeritus of Psychiatry at the University of Western Ontario in London, Ontario and continues an active clinical practice in the treatment of patients with chronic pain.

He has been very prolific in researching various aspects of pain, dementia, and psychiatric problems, such as dissociative identity disorder and hysteria. Dr. Merskey published over three hundred fifty scientific papers and was selected by Dr. John Bonica as the first chair of the Committee on Classifications of Pain from the International Association for the Study of Pain. He has been actively involved in this international association and its prestigious journal, *Pain*, for many years and is the founding editor-in-chief of the *Journal of the Canadian Pain Society, Pain Research and Management.*

Dr. Merskey is also well-known for his clinical work. He is extremely knowledgeable, as you would expect from his scientific achievements. He is also very compassionate and a tireless advocate for his patients.

Russel Portenoy, MD

Dr. Portenoy received his medical training from the Maryland School of Medicine and further training in neurology at the Albert Einstein College of Medicine. Currently, he is the Chairman of the Department of Medicine and Palliative Care at Beth Israel Medical Center. He also continues as a Professor of Neurology at the Albert Einstein College of Medicine, is editor-in-chief of the journal *Pain and Symptom Management*, and an associate editor for the journal *Pain.*

Dr. Portenoy has lead a very productive research career. His research interests involve mainly the management and treatment of cancer pain and pain in patients with AIDS. He received many awards, including the American Pain Society's Wilbert Fordyce Award for Lifetime Excellence and Clinical Investigation and the American Pain Society's Distinguished Service Award.

Dennis Turk, Ph.D.

Dr. Turk was born in New York in 1946. His undergraduate training was at the University of Florida under the supervision of Dr. Donald Meichenbaum. He obtained a doctorate in clinical psychology from the University of Waterloo, Ontario and held the position of professor at several universities, including Yale University and the University of Pittsburgh. He currently holds the prestigious position of John and Emma Bonica Professorship in Anesthesiology and Pain Research through the University of Washington. He is also the Director of the Fibromyalgia Research Center.

Widely recognized for his scientific work, especially related to how physical, psychological, and social aspects of pain all work together, Dr. Turk has discovered important innovations for the assessment and treatment of pain. He has investigated psychological aspects of pain management and pain programs, and helped explain the complexities of assessing and treating various chronic pain conditions. He was awarded the Janet Travell Award for outstanding contributions to the field of pain from the American Academy of Pain Management. In addition to his many scientific articles and books, he is currently the editor-in-chief of the *Clinical Journal of Pain.*

Patrick Wall, DM

Dr. Wall was born in Nottingham, England, earned his graduate degrees in medicine from Oxford University, and held numerous faculty appointments in the areas of physiology and anatomy at universities, such as Yale University, Harvard, Massachusetts Institute of Technology, and the University of Chicago. His last position, before his death a few years ago, was as Professor Emeritus at the University of London. He won numerous awards in recognition of his research work in pain. He was also a founding member of the International Association for the Study of Pain and a founding editor of the journal *Pain.*

Dr. Wall had a wide range of research interests, but most specifically, he was focused on the physical and sensory mechanisms responsible for how pain is transmitted throughout the body. He published widely, with scientific articles and books. Several of his books were co-authored with Dr. Ronald Melzack. As discussed under the section for Dr. Melzack, Dr. Wall was instrumental with Dr. Melzack in developing the revolutionary gate control theory of pain.

Clifford Woolf, MD, Ph.D.

Dr. Woolf received both his medical training and a Ph.D. in physiology from the University of Witwatersrand in Johannesburg, South Africa, plus a Masters degree from the Harvard Medical School, and post doctoral training under the supervision of Dr. Patrick Wall. Dr. Woolf holds the prestigious Richard J. Kitz Professorship in Anesthesiology Research at the Harvard Medical School and Massachusetts General Hospital. He has numerous awards for his work on pain and is currently an associate editor of the *Journal of Neuroscience.*

His main research interests have involved investigations into how pain mechanisms work, including sensory changes after nerve damage and changes in sensory neurons after inflammation. Dr. Woolf is widely recognized for his major contributions to understanding the mechanisms of central sensitization. This occurs when body pain creates changes in a person's brain, which then makes the individual more sensitive to pain. He has been able to show how this process contributes to persistent pain. He has been active in taking these basic research steps further, in looking at how analgesia can be used to help prevent central sensitization in patients with persistent pain.

Discussion

As noted, earlier, much of the information from this chapter has been taken from the following article: "Profiles and Perspectives of the Leading Contributors in the Field of Pain." This article was published in 2001 and is found in *The Pain Clinic,* the journal from the World Society of Pain Clinicians. The authors were all from the University of Regina: Gordon Asmundson, Thomas Hadjistavropoulos, and Miranda Antonishyn.

Recognition of the top pain scientists in the world is an important contribution. These authors then took their survey a step further and asked each of these top scientists for their ideas about where the research in the field of pain is heading. Most of the scientists were very enthusiastic about the growth of research in the field of pain and excited about how much progress has been made. Dr. Portenoy stated: "Pain research is in an extraordinary vibrant period." Dr. Turk said: "There has been an explosion of interest and research in the assessment, treatment, and rehabilitation of people with pain." According to Dr. Woolf, "Pain research is in the midst of very rapid progress" (Asmundson et al., 2001).

Several of the top scientists emphasized similar themes and recommendations. It was felt that pain research needed to combine very basic scientific research with clinical research into the best methods to assess and treat patients in pain. Basic scientific research is necessary to understand the underlying physiological and biological mechanisms of pain. To do that, it is necessary to combine the work from many disciplines, including medicine, pharmacology, anatomy, physiology, psychology, genetics, and nursing. These and other clinical specialties all provide unique knowledge that needs to be combined together to produce a more detailed understanding of pain and better treatments for the people who are suffering.

Many of the top scientists stated that more government funding needs to be devoted toward this type of integrated pain research. It was emphasized that clinical providers – of all specialties – need more basic education into the complexities and the details of the treatment of pain. The International Association for the Study of Pain has been a leading advocate of this kind of increased education and training.

All the top scientists were very optimistic about the incredible discoveries that have been made, especially over recent years. More and more research funding is being devoted toward pain research. The education of doctors – and all clinical providers – has increased and gradually more and more treatments are becoming available to help people with long-term and chronic pain.

• • •

Sarah did not understand all the details about how these top scientists went about their scientific work. Even the descriptions of their work were often beyond her. What she did take from this article and from the discussion among the scientists was their dedication and commitment to the field of pain and their hope for how this research has been growing and even exploding to the benefit of all people in pain. She needed to hear this type of hope. In her Website she hoped that she could convey some of this promise and commitment.

Part Four:

Learning from a Great Pain Society

CHAPTER ONE

The International Association for the Study of Pain (IASP)

It all started in a convent – in 1973 in Issaquah, Washington, about forty miles from Seattle. In this hallowed setting, Dr. John Bonica proposed the creation of the International Association for the Study of Pain. This organization was a longtime dream for Dr. Bonica. Throughout the years, his vision and tireless efforts developed this organization. It has continued to flourish to this day.

Dr. Bonica and the IASP have had some special help from Louisa Jones. She was the first employee, became the executive secretary, and has devoted thirty-two years of her life to the IASP. A recent book, *The Paths of Pain*, was dedicated to her skill, integrity, wisdom, and unfailing commitment. (More about this book and IASP can be found in the Epilogue.)

IASP is truly a multidisciplinary organization. This is one of the keys to its effectiveness and part of Dr. Bonica's dream. Every professional who is willing to offer knowledge, education, or clinical care about pain has something to offer the organization and has been encouraged to join. In turn, the organization has a mandate to offer something of value, not only to these professionals, but toward a future for better research and treatment for people in pain.

Education is the backbone of change. This is a founding belief for this international organization. After all, what is the point of developing new treatments if no one knows about them or knows how to use them properly? For this reason, IASP has developed educational materials and a pain curriculum for all healthcare professionals. These courses are updated frequently and help professionals from all disciplines learn about the fundamentals, as well as the new developments in the field of pain research, diagnosis, treatment, and prevention.

Detailed research-based education about pain is often missing in many disciplines, even in medicine. Future doctors are taught about injuries, illnesses, and treatments, but often lack a thorough understanding of pain itself. This is what sparked the development of this international organization in the first place. As IASP has emphasized over the years, it is important to treat not only the underlying cause of pain, but also to help patients with the pain itself. This is especially true for chronic pain conditions.

The International Association for the Study of Pain is organized into over sixty chapters in countries throughout the world. Each chapter has a national organization with the same goals as the IASP: education and the promotion of a greater understanding and treatment for people who suffer with pain. Each country or chapter holds an annual scientific meeting and, in some cases, there are joint meetings between chapters. Many of the chapters also publish their own scientific journal.

One of the main benefits of IASP, for patients and scientists alike, is the publication of their prestigious journal, *Pain.* This is the leading journal in the pain field. This journal was first published in January of 1975 and has grown in size since then. Currently it publishes monthly issues. There are also supplements and additional scientific publications distributed by IASP, including ethical guidelines for investigations of experimental pain and standards for physicians in training.

In 1987, IASP was granted a special designation with the World Health Organization. The association was granted status as a non-governmental organization (NGO), closely affiliated with the World Health Organization. The IASP counsel also has a special concern for individuals in developing countries, who experience difficulties finding adequate pain treatment. Several programs have been established to promote pain education, knowledge, and treatments in these developing countries. Some IASP chapters have adopted members from developing countries to help them develop programs. There is also an Adopt a University Library program, which helps libraries in developing countries gain access to free membership to research journals on pain, and access to university medical libraries in larger, more developed countries.

IASP holds a world congress every three years. These have been ongoing since the first world congress in

Florence, Italy in 1975. These high-level scientific meetings occur in glamorous places throughout the world including Paris, Vancouver, Edinburgh, Italy, and Australia, as examples.

A detailed history of the International Association for the Study of Pain, the American Pain Society, and the Intractable Pain Society of Great Britain are described and documented in the History of Pain Collection at UCLA. This amazing collection is highlighted in the next chapter.

CHAPTER TWO

The History of Pain Project (UCLA)

In 1993, Dr. John Liebeskind began this project by audiotaping interviews with leaders and pioneers in the pain field. He asked about the details of their research, their views on where the field of pain research has been, and where it is headed. Now there are over sixty-five personal accounts preserved in this collection. Some of the giants interviewed in this field include doctors and scientists, namely, John Bonica, Patrick Wall, Ronald Melzack, Jean-Murray Besson, Michael Cousins, Ronald Dubner, Kathleen Foley, Jan Gybels, Ulf Lindblom, John Loeser, Harold Merskey, and Paolo Procacci. Soon these oral histories will become available as CDs.

Dr. Marcia Meldrum is a medical historian and has taken over the work from Dr. Liebeskind, following his death in 1997. Archivist Russell Johnson also carries on Liebeskind's work. In a recent article about this collection, Dr. Meldrum discussed the privilege and honor that Dr. Liebeskind felt in doing this collection. He felt privileged to have witnessed the coming together of doctors and scientists from many different fields, in different countries, working toward a common goal to learn about pain and to help people who suffer from pain. This collection is an incredibly impressive project. It is now called the John C. Liebeskind History of Pain Collection at the University of California, Los Angeles (UCLA).

The Liebeskind Collection started out with interviews of notable scientists in the pain research field. It has gone on to collect papers and records from pain associations and societies around the world. Personal papers, letters, and records about these scientists and their lives are included. These records help us see what was involved in some of the early work in this vast field of pain research. These documents include some of the early letters between Dr. John Bonica and Dr. Patrick Wall, as they planned the first International Association for the Study of Pain meeting. There are records and hand-drawings of twelve hundred nerve injury patients treated during World War II. There are original copies of pain journals from Chile and China. Also included are the first issues of the bulletin of the Nigerian Society for the Study of Pain (1998); programs and brochures from Portugal's First National Day of Struggle Against Pain (1999); and photographs, brochures, and chapter histories of more than thirty-six ISAP member countries. This collection even includes the tape of a song, *Over Pain We'll Be Victorious*, written by New Zealander Dr. Bob Large for the 1990 IASP symposium.

As Suzanne read about the History of Pain Collection, she was moved by how these scientists had devoted their lives to the study of pain. These were scientists from all over the world, working together to find cures and new treatments for the millions of people in pain.

Marni Jackson was also moved when she visited the History of Pain Collection in Los Angeles as part of the research for her book, *Pain: The Fifth Vital Sign*, published in 2002. This impressive book presents an understanding of pain from a writer and journalist's point of view. Jackson is a migraine sufferer; this research and visit to Los Angeles had special meaning for her.

The Liebeskind Collection is located in the History and Special Collections Department of the Louise M. Darling Biomedical Library at the University of California, Los Angeles. During her visit, Jackson met Russell Johnson, one of the co-directors of this collection. With Johnson's help, Jackson delved into the work of a famous American physician, Dr. Silas Weir Mitchell. As a writer, Jackson was particularly intrigued, not only by Dr. Mitchell's work as a famous neurologist, but also by the fact that he was a poet. Jackson noted in her book, that at the height of Dr. Mitchell's fame in the 1870s, he was as celebrated for his novels and poetry as he was for his medical and surgical work. She had a chance to review a book he wrote called *Gunshot Wounds and Other Injuries of Nerves.* It chronicled detailed case studies of Dr. Mitchell's treatment of soldiers injured in the Civil War (Mitchell, 1872). These investigations were vivid and helped explain the different types of pain and nerve damage that occurred with injuries from war. This amazing research helped form the foundation of how we understand nerve pain and neurosurgery today.

In 1904, Dr. Mitchell wrote a fascinating book called *Doctor and Patient.* Jackson offered some quotes from this book in hers, such as "There are very few instances of chronic ailments, however slight which should not be met by advice as to modes of living" (Mitchell, 1904; in Jackson, 2002). Even back in 1904, a famous neurologist and surgeon wrote that the treatment for chronic pain should involve medical treatments and assistance to the patient on how to cope with the general stresses of living.

When Suzanne discovered this quote in Jackson's book, it sent a shudder down her spine. This is exactly what the counselors were preaching to her in the chronic pain program. She saw evidence for the effectiveness of this idea in her own life. One of the main turning points for her was the start of part-time work at the dental clinic. This not only helped to boost her confidence and reduce her stress, but it improved her capacity for coping with her chronic pain. Dr. Mitchell discovered this truth in his work with soldiers suffering from nerve damage following gunshots in war. These same ideas are used today in multidisciplinary chronic pain programs; it is the same kind of program where Suzanne, Ashley, Mike, and Sarah were helped.

As Dr. Meldrum is aware, it is not possible for everyone to visit UCLA and the Liebeskind Collection. To spread the word, she presents talks and papers about the history of pain throughout the world. Dr. Meldrum has also collaborated on research projects involving the history of cancer pain, has published papers in medical journals, and helped set up a Website for the Liebeskind Collection.

This History of Pain Project is a fascinating one. The subject is complex and the characters and scientists throughout its history are colorful and insightful. We all owe a great debt of gratitude to Dr. Liebeskind for his devotion in establishing this collection, which will benefit us all.

• • •

The John C. Liebeskind History of Pain Collection
Website is located at:

www.library.ucla.edu/libraries/biomed/his/pain.html

Marni Jackson's book, *Pain: The Fifth Vital Sign* was published by Random House Canada in 2002. An alternate name for this book is *Pain: The Science and Culture of Why We Hurt.*

Epilogue

WE HAVE COME A LONG, LONG WAY

When you look back, you can see just how far you have come. Looking back (and forward) is just what several prominent doctors and scientists have done in the field of pain. Their thoughts and ideas have been organized into a fascinating book, *The Paths of Pain* (2005).

Dr. Harold Merskey, Dr. John Loeser, and Dr. Ronald Dubner, editors of this book, have brought together forty-nine international pain experts to write about the remarkable progress that has been made. There are chapters on neck, back, migraine, cancer, and fibromyalgia pain. Other experts have discussed the measurement of pain, brain imaging studies, and new forms of neurological, pharmacological, and multidisciplinary types of treatment.

One area of rapid growth has involved the use of brain scans, such as Magnetic Resonance Imaging (MRI) and Positron Emission Tomography (PET). Dr. Catharine Bushnell, from the Centre for Research on Pain at McGill University, has summarized this research on brain imaging in her chapter entitled, "Brain Imaging of Pain" (Bushnell, 2005). She writes about the thirty-year history of this field, but notes, interestingly, that the vast majority of studies have been done within the past five years. This field is now at the point where it is expanding rapidly. As Dr. Bushnell says, brain imaging studies are growing at an exponential rate. Undoubtedly, this is one of the fastest growing areas of pain research.

Scientists are learning more each day about how the different parts of the brain influence the pain you experience. For example, when you suffer from a shoulder injury, pain signals are sent back and forth between your shoulder, spinal cord, and certain parts of your brain. "The body detects and the brain reacts," is how the famous neuroscientist and pain researcher, Dr. Patrick Wall, describes it. The spinal cord acts like a bridge for signals coming and going between your injured body and your brain (Wall, 2000).

Scientists are making some incredible progress in understanding how the pain system works. Dr. Charles Vierck, a neuroscientist from the University of Florida, wrote a detailed review of this research in a recent article published in the prestigious journal, *Pain (2006).* He explained how fibromyalgia (a form of chronic pain) usually follows from an initial injury to the body. Persistent pain from this injury involves signals sent to the brain, which can change how the brain works. The brain then sends out signals, which cause pain to be experienced in other areas of the body. Poor sleep, fatigue, and high levels of stress follow. Changes to the brain can also lead to the body's increased sensitivity, which leads to an even higher level of pain spread throughout the body. These brain changes and patterns have been described by Melzack in his neuromatrix model (Melzack, 2001; Melzack and Katz, 2006). Additional stresses, such as the inability to work, can make this situation all the worse, resulting in even higher pain levels.

There has been an incredible amount of research in this area. "Voluminous," says Dr. Vierck. I have purposely simplified this technical research to make it easy to read. If you have the strength to read the scientific details, though, you will learn just how complicated and amazing this research is. A reference to this review article by Dr. Vierck is included in the reference list at the end of this book.

Brain imaging and fibromyalgia are not the only areas of pain research to see such growth. In fact, the whole field has shown great gains. For example, looking back at the early days of general anesthesia to prevent the pain from surgery, you can see an illustration of just how far we have come.

Dr. Scott Fishman and Lisa Berger, in their book, *The War on Pain* (2000), provide a colorful illustration of this miraculous technique. In the Massachusett General Hospital's original operating room, called the Etherdome, the first surgery using ether as a general anesthetic was performed by William Morton. He was a dentist who performed an operation involving the removal of a tumor in the lower jaw of a twenty-year-old patient. William Morton administered the ether, while the hospital's leading surgeon, Dr. John Collins Warner, performed the surgical procedure.

> "As Warner began his first incision, the entire operating theater fell silent. It was as if everyone was holding his breath, waiting for a cry of pain from the patient. But he was in a deep sleep, even as blood from severed arteries spurted out. Within minutes, Dr. Warner had removed the mass from the bloody jaw and Abbott (the

> patient) was still unconscious. Dr. Warner's assistant sewed up and bandaged the incision, then waited for Abbott to regain consciousness." (Fishman & Berger, 2000, page 28)

Then another famous Harvard surgeon, Dr. W.J. Bigelow chimed in from his seat in the audience. "Our craft has, once and for all, has been robbed of its terrors," (Fishman & Berger, 2000, page 28).

Fishman and Berger have a colorful way of describing these and other dramas in the history of pain. For example, before this discovery of ether, whiskey was often the preferred anesthetic. "Surgeons were known to enter the operating room with a bottle of whiskey in each hand – one for the patient and one for the doctor so he could endure his patient's screams" (2000, page 29).

Since that time, many new pain medications have been developed. Yet, as Fishman and Berger describe, "The gold standard of pain relief is still old-fashioned opiates" (2000). Opioid is the general name of the drug, natural or synthetic, that acts to reduce pain. Dr. Fishman is an anesthesiologist and lists in his book the types of medications that fall into this category. Morphine and heroin were two of the first opioid painkillers. Other variations include:

- Codeine (one-sixth as strong as morphine)
- Meperidine (known as Demerol)
- Methodone (developed during World War II as a substitute for hard-to-get morphine)

- Hydromorphone (now known as Dilaudid, ten times stronger than morphine)
- Fentanyl (the only opioid used in a patch form on the skin) (Fishman and Berger, 2000, page 311)

Despite these early discoveries, it has only been recently that doctors and scientists have figured out exactly how these pain medications work. Dr. Patrick Wall, in his book *Pain: The Science of Suffering (2000),* described how these amazing discoveries happened. First, Dr. Tony Yaksh from the United States found two areas – one in the middle of the brain and the other in a spinal cord where pain messages arrived from the injured area of a person's body. Next, Dr. Kosterlitz, from Aberdeen, Scotland, discovered that the brain itself is able to produce its own narcotic-like substances. These are called endorphins. These pain-killing substances from a person's own brain can be produced even in the absence of any medication. When pain-killing medicine is given to a person, it travels to the brain and stimulates the part of the brain that can create these endorphins. Pain medications work on special receptors that we all have, which react specifically to natural and synthetic opioids. These were amazing discoveries and have happened only within the past twenty years.

It was a surprising discovery to find out that the body makes its own narcotics – endorphins – and has receptors to react to them. These naturally occurring substances can fight pain. When these findings from various scientists were put together, it became clear that morphine and other painkillers imitate and enhance part of what the body is already accomplishing to fight pain. Opioid medication is able to combine with the body's own pain-killing substances and, in combination, can reduce pain as well as other reactions such as anxiety and hormone responses.

Scientists have since discovered that cannabis works the same way. It has been found that the brain itself produces cannabis-like substances. There are special cells in the brain that react specifically to natural and synthetic cannabis. This has helped scientists and doctors to understand how cannabis can be useful in treating certain types of pain.

Understanding how medications work is a lot more complicated than has been described in this chapter. It is mind-boggling to learn about what really happens in the brain on a molecular and chemical level. This early research was truly groundbreaking, though. These amazing discoveries have helped scientists and doctors to find new ways and new substances that can provide more effective relief for pain. An incredible amount of work is being done all over the world. This work starts with basic research, on a microscopic level, into how pain signals and pain pathways function. New molecules, chemicals, and cells are being discovered, which play a central role in the development and maintenance of persistent pain.

One of the obstacles for research today is the difficulty for scientists to keep abreast of the many different types of molecules being discovered. The good news is there are so many possibilities (or "targets" as the scientists say) for effective pain treatments. In fact, Dr. Allan Basbaum has described this situation as an explosion of targets. Or phrased another way, "lots of targets, not enough arrows" (Basbaum, 2005, page, 516). Currently, doctors endeavor to find the best medication to treat each specific injury or illness that may be causing the pain experienced by an individual. But, individuals – even with the same injuries – respond differently to different types of medications. In the future, doctors and scientists are hoping to find the best medication, not only for each particular injury, but also for each particular individual with that injury.

As wonderful new medications become more available to help people in pain, new challenges are created. Some obvious concerns regarding medications include the threat of addictions, substance abuse, and the non-medical or recreational use of pain medications. Government agencies are clamping down and monitoring doctors' practices. This has put a lot of heat on doctors who are already feeling pressure from their patients' need for help. "A collision between the War on Drugs and the War on Pain," is how Fishman and Berger have described this situation (2000). They call it a "perfect storm of controversy." Doctors are caught in the middle. Some are frightened of legal ramifications if they prescribe too much pain medication – or being sued by their patients if they don't prescribe enough. Some patients are losing out and not receiving the help they need.

Sometimes this war is fuelled by sensational media reports. The media can spread negative stereotypes about people with chronic pain, or individuals who need pain medication to treat their pain. For example, many patients with chronic pain are helped by the long-acting opioid: Oxycontin. This relatively new medication has also become popular among recreational drug users. Some rural areas near Appalachia, Virginia suffered such a rise in the illegal use of Oxycontin, that the medication was sensationalized as "hillbilly heroin" (Tough, 2001). This term added to doctors' fears in prescribing Oxycontin and patients fears of taking it for their pain. Unfortunately, few people read enough of the fine print to know the details. Experienced drug users were getting a heroin-like high from Oxycontin by crushing the pills, then injecting or snorting them. This is not how people in pain use this medication under the guidance of their doctors. Yet, the fear and stigma persist. (Millroy, 2001; Tough, 2001)

On a more positive note, drug advertising, of all things, has been a great help for sufferers of fibromyalgia. The drug company Pfizer has started marketing a new medication for fibromyalgia on television. Near the end of the television commercial, a woman turns to the camera and says in a serious tone, "Fibromyalgia is a real, widespread pain condition." Although this is a paid advertisement, it does offer a voice of validation for millions of people in pain. Alex Berenson, from the New York Times, offered a reaction from Lynne Matallana. As president of the National Fibromyalgia Association, she said new drugs, such as Lyrica (and its television commercial) would help people accept the existence of fibromyalgia. Mr. Berenson quoted Ms. Matallana as saying, "The day that the FDA approved a drug and we had a public service announcement, my pain became real to people" (Berenson, 2008).

Doctors and patients need clear guidelines to deal with the War on Pain and the War on Drugs. A balanced approach was recommended by a panel of experts in a recent meeting in 2007, sponsored by the American Pain Foundation. This group of scientists and doctors also emphasized the serious problems of under-treatment for individuals with chronic pain. The expert panel concluded that:

> "Pain affects more Americans than diabetes, heart disease, and cancer combined. Now is the time to build consensus on pain management and opioid use in America and drive perceptions toward a more balanced view. Alleviating pain in patients with legitimate medical needs remains a medical imperative" (American Pain Foundation, April 2008).

Pain medications continue to provide a huge benefit to millions of people with chronic or long-term pain. While this is helpful, it is not really what individuals in pain want. People in pain want a cure. They want a total and permanent end to their suffering – a chance to return to a normal life. Several years ago, doctors and scientists from Australia took a big step in this direction.

In 1997, Dr. Barbara Wallis, Dr. Susan Lord, and Dr. Nikolai Bogduk published an incredible research paper in the prestigious journal, *Pain*. This paper provided further evidence for the usefulness of a new neurosurgery technique for patients with chronic neck (whiplash) pain. This surgical technique involved placing an electrode, under local anesthesia, near spinal nerves in the patient's neck. A radio frequency electrode was then used to create lesions in the spinal nerves, which were causing the patient's chronic neck pain. Of the nine patients who received the neurosurgical treatment, six experienced complete relief of their pain.

This preliminary research by Drs. Wallis, Lord, and Bogduk is fascinating on many levels. First, it provides further evidence for a promising new surgery technique to help people with chronic neck pain. The authors state clearly that this operation does not provide a permanent cure, yet pain relief can last for months or even years in some patients (1997).

This research also provides further evidence that whiplash pain is caused by damage to a particular joint in the spine (cervical zygapophyseal joint). Earlier findings from this research group showed that damage to this spinal joint could be the cause of long-term neck pain (caused by whiplash injuries) in about fifty percent of patients. As reviewed by Wallis, Lord and Bogduk (1997), These findings highlight the real and physical nature of chronic pain and help pinpoint an exact area of the neck for treatments to be targeted.

Drs. Wallis, Lord, and Bogduk then emphasize yet another benefit of their research. They showed that when all of a patient's pain is taken away, the patient's psychological distress disappears as well. If chronic pain were caused in any way by psychological factors, this would not occur. This research shows, quite clearly, that it is the physical pain (and related losses) that cause psychological stress, not the opposite.

New advances in technology, such as the radio frequency surgical technology discussed above, are also devoted to making pain treatments more accurate and more precise. Part of this technology involves the development of new medications. (Drugs that work like smart bombs, according to Fishman and Berger, 2000, page 260.) Another important part involves new techniques to identify specific nerve pathways and even single nerves that can be altered to reduce the pain experienced. Dr. Fishman predicts: "The tools I use to silence nerve pathways will become so exact that I will be able to pinpoint single nerves – a micro-strand smaller than a human hair – and deliver a drop of medication, a nanosecond of heat, or a blip of electricity to an individual nerve cell anywhere in the human anatomy." (Fishman and Berger, 2000, page 259)

Future techniques will be done through the use of lasers, microprocessors, and fiber optics that can guide the steady hand of robotics into the tangled web of nerves and delicate brain tissue, which may be responsible for an individual's pain. Fishman and Berger (2000) discuss one of the latest medical tools. A laser is placed through a small hole in the skin and guided with a tiny video camera into a slipped or herniated disc in the back to surgically repair a problem. Such treatments are still experimental. Yet, there is the potential for doctors to be able to perform major surgery, deep within the body, with little or no risk to the patient.

In the future, these techniques will be enhanced much further by sophisticated imaging instruments, which will allow doctors to see clearly inside the body and its areas of painful injury. Even today, these imaging technologies are becoming more useful and more powerful. New tools like functional MRIs have been developed, for example. They are able to generate pictures of the brain and the body that are not yet completely understood. It takes time for researchers to become familiar with the new technologies being developed. First, scientists learn how to see more clearly (inside the body). Then, they need to understand exactly what it is that they are seeing. Better pictures of the brain and the body will help doctors and scientists to understand more about the causes of pain, and ultimately fine-tune the treatments necessary for much needed cures.

These new scientific findings and technologies for pain treatment will go a long way toward helping to reduce and eliminate the pain and suffering for millions of people. This is an important goal. It is also important to help individuals in pain reduce the losses and suffering that follow from their injuries and persistent pain. Psychological and rehabilitative treatments can provide significant benefits in this area. Doctors are also busy researching how multidisciplinary treatment programs can help, not only with an individual's pain, but also help to diminish the losses and life disruption that often accompanies long-term pain.

Suzanne, Ashley, Sarah, and Mike were treated in a multidisciplinary hospital pain program. This program helped them to reduce their pain, to reduce their stress, and to find ways to move forward in their lives. As they started putting these ideas into effect, they realized that reductions in stress, even the stresses caused by their pain, helped to reduce their flare-ups and their overall level of pain. They realized that taking active steps to regain control over their lives helped to reduce some of these stresses and, in turn, helped to lessen their pain.

It has been a difficult journey for Suzanne, Ashley, Mike, and Sarah. They still hope that, someday, they may be able to live without pain. They have learned a lot, though. They continue to learn. And, year-by-year, their pain lessens and they feel more and more in control of their lives. Now, at least, they have lives to lead.

Whenever she could, Sarah would send news of her new discoveries to Suzanne, Mike, and Ashley. Sarah has come a long way from her darkest days. Hope was now possible.

"Back when we first met, in the green hallway of that old hospital, we never thought that any of this could ever happen," wrote Suzanne, in one of her many emails back to Sarah.

"Yes," wrote Ashley. "It has been truly unbelievable."

Internet Resources

American Academy of Pain Medicine. **www.painmed.org**

American Headache Society. **www.ahsnet.org**

American Pain Foundation. **www.painfoundation.org**

American Pain Society. **www.ampainsoc.org**

Brainstorm. American Headache Society. **www.ahsnet.org/brainstorm.php**

Canadian Pain Society. **www.canadianpainsociety.ca**

Decade of Pain Task Force. American Pain Society, American Pain Foundation, American Academy of Pain Medicine, and the American Headache Society. **www.decadeofpain.org**

Fibromyalgia Network. **www.fmnetwork.com**

Fifth Vital Sign campaign. American Pain Society. **www.ampainsoc.org/advocacy**

For Grace: The Dream of Never Again. **www.forgrace.org**

The John C. Liebeskind History of Pain Collection. University of California, Los Angeles. **www.library.ucla.edu/libraries/biomed/his/pain.html**

Lifting the Burden. World Health Organization.
www.who.int
(access through "headache" in Website's search engine)

My Pain. National Pain Foundation.
www.nationalpainfoundation.org

National Pain Foundation.
www.nationalpainfoundation.org

Pain and the law. For persons in pain. The Center for Health Law Studies at St. Louis University and The American Society of Law, Medicine and Ethics.
www.painandthelaw.org

Pain Care Coalition. American Pain Society.
www.ampainsoc.org/advocacy

Pain Care Minutes. American Pain Society.
www.ampainsoc.org

Pain Explained (painexplained.ca) campaign. Canadian Pain Society and Canadian Pain Coalition.
www.painexplained.ca

The Patient Pain Manifesto. Canadian Pain Society.
www.canadianpainsociety.ca/newsandannouncements

Power Over Pain. American Pain Foundation.
www.painfoundation.org

PubMed Website: **www.ncbi.nlm.nih.gov/pubmed**

The physician's voice in pain medicine. American Academy of Pain Medicine. **www.painmed.org**

Untying the Knot. National Pain Foundation and the Academy of Pain Medicine. **www.nationalpainfoundation.org/untyingtheknot.html**

Voices of the people. American Pain Foundation. **www.painfoundation.org**

Women in Pain Initiative. For Grace: The Dream of Never Again. **www.forgrace.org**

World Headache Alliance. **www.w-h-a.org**

World Health Organization. **www.who.int**

Books on Chronic Pain and Fibromylagia

Bowers, K.S. (1983). *Hypnosis for the seriously curious.* New York: Norton.

Caudill, M. and Benson, H. (2008). *Managing pain before it manages you. Third Edition.* New York: Guilford Press.

Fishman, S. and Berger, L. (2000). *The war on pain.* New York: HarperCollins Publishers.

Jackson, M. (2002). *Pain: The fifth vital sign.* Toronto: Random House Canada. (an alternate name of this book is *Pain: The science and culture of why we hurt)*

Lynch, M. (2003). *Surviving your personal injuries, claim and litigation: A Guide Book.* Halifax, Nova Scotia: Dalhousie Health Sciences. (Available through the Dalhousie Health Sciences Bookstore (telephone: 903-494-6701 or email susan.kingston@dal.ca))

Melzack, R. and Wall, P. (1996). *The challenge of pain.* London, England: Penguin Books.

Pellegrino, M.L. (1996). *Understanding post-traumatic fibromyalgia.* Columbus, Ohio: Anadem Publications.

Pellegrino, M.L. (2005). *Fibromyalgia: Up close and personal.* Columbus, Ohio: Anadem Publications.

Starlanyl, D. (1999). *The fibromyalgia advocate.* Oakland, California: New Harbinger Publications.

Sternbach, R.A. (1987). *Mastering pain.* Toronto, Ontario. Random House.

Turk, D.C. and Winter, F. (2006). *The pain survival guide.* Washington, DC. American Psychological Association.

Wall, P. (2000). *The science of suffering.* New York: Columbia University Press.

Scientific and Media References

American Medical Association. (1993). *Guides to the evaluation of permanent impairment, 4th Edition.* Chicago, Illinois: *American Medical Association.*

American Pain Foundation. (April 2008). *Provider prescribing patterns and perceptions: Identifying solutions to build consensus on opioid use in pain management – A roundtable discussion. www.painfoundation.org.*

Asmundson, G., Hadjistavropoulos, T. and Antonishyn, M. (2001). Profiles and perspectives of the leading contributors in the field of pain. *The Pain Clinic 13*(1): 55–69.

Basbaum, A.I. (2005). The future of pain therapy: Something old, something new, something borrowed, something blue. In H. Merskey, J.D. Loeser, and R. Dubner (Eds.) *The paths of pain: 1975–2005.* Seattle, Washington: IASP Press.

Berenson, A. (2008). Drug approved. Is disease real? January 14, 2008. www.nytimes.com.

Bowers, K.S. (1983). *Hypnosis for the seriously curious.* New York: Norton.

Brennan, F. and Cousins, M. (2004). Pain relief is a human right. *Pain: Clinical Updates* September. Seattle, Washington: International Association for the Study of Pain.

Bushnell, C. (2005). Brain imaging of pain. In H. Merskey, J.D. Loeser, and R. Dubner (Eds.) *The paths of pain: 1975–2005.* Seattle, Washington: IASP Press.

Campbell, J. (1995). Pain: *The fifth vital sign: Advocacy and policy.* Presidential Address to the American Pain Society. Los Angeles, California: American Pain Society. www.ampainsoc.org/advocacy/fifth.html

Cheek, D.B. and LeCron, L.M. (1968). *Clinical hypnotherapy.* New York: Grune and Stratton.

Chronic Pain Initiative. (2000). *Report of the chair of chronic pain panels.* Toronto, Ontario: Workplace Safety and Insurance Board.

Chronic Pain Initiative. (2000). *Report of the chronic pain expert advisory panel.* Toronto, Ontario: Workplace Safety and Insurance Board.

Chronic Pain Initiative. (2000). *Report of the chronic pain policy advisory panel.* Toronto, Ontario: Workplace Safety and Insurance Board.

Cohen, S.B. (1980). Editorial: Being one's own anesthesiologist. *The American Journal of Clinical Hypnosis 22(*3): 121–123.

Copenhagen Declaration. (1992). Myopain '92. Abstracts from the Second World Congress on Myofascial Pain and Fibromyalgia. *Scandanavian Journal of Rheumatology, 94 Supplement* 1-70. (no authors listed)

Dozois, D. (2009). An interview with Dr. Ronald Melzack. *Psynopsis, Winter, 2.*

Duckworth, M., Iezzi, T. and Donohue, W.T. (2008).

Motor vehicle accidents: Medical, psychosocial and legal consequences. San Diego, CA: Academic Press. Duersing, L. (2004). Pain management advocacy: From the one to the many. *Pain Community News, Fall: 1 & 4.*Fishman, S. and Berger, L. (2000). *The war on pain.* New York: HarperCollins Publishers.

Gatchel, R. (2005). *Clinical essentials of pain management.* Washington, DC: American Psychological Association.

Gatchel, R., Peng, Y., Peters, M., Fuchs, P. and Turk, D. (2007). The biopsychosocial approach to chronic pain: Scientific advances and future directions. *Pain 133(*4): 581–624.

Gowers, A. (1904). A lecture on lumbago: lessons and analogues. *British Medical Journal, 1, 117-12.* (cited in Moldofsky and Merskey, 2005)

Gureje, O., Simon, G. and Von Korff, M. (2001). A cross-sectional study of the course of persistent pain in primary care. *Pain 92:* 195–200.

Gureje, O., Von Korff, M., Simon, G. and Gater, R. (1998). Persistent pain and well-being: A world health original study in primary care. *Journal of the American Medical Association 280*(7): 147–151.

Hercz, R. (2000). Surgery without anesthetic: The outer limits of hypnosis. *Toronto Life,* Fall, supplement.

Jackson, M. (2002). *Pain: The fifth vital sign:* Toronto: Random House Canada. (an alternate name for this book is *Pain: The science and culture of why we hurt)*

Johnston, C. (2001). The patient pain manifesto. *Canadian Pain Society.* www.canadianpainsociety.ca/newsandannouncements.

Kirsch, I., and Lynn, S. J. (1995). The altered state of hypnosis: Changes in the theoretical landscape. *American Psychologist 50:* 846–858.

Kuch, K. (2000). Psychological factors in chronic pain and chronic pain disability. In *Chronic Pain Initiative: Report of the chronic pain expert panel.* Toronto, Ontario: Workplace Safety and Insurance Board.

Lang, E.S., Berbaum, K.S., Faintuch, S., Hatsiopoulou, O., Halsey, N., Li, X., Berbaum, M.L., Laser, E. and Baum, J. (2006). Adjuctive self-hypnotic relaxation for outpatient medical procedures: A prospective randomized trial with women undergoing large core breast biopsy. *Pain 126: 155–164.*

Melzack, R. (2001). Pain and the neuromatrix in the brain. *Journal of Dental Education* 65(12), 1378-1382.

Melzack, R. and Katz, J. (2006). Pain in the 21st century: The neuromatrix and beyond. In G. Young, A.W. Kane, and K. Nicholson (Eds.) Psychological knowledge in court. New York: Springer Science-Business Media Inc.

Merskey, H. (2005). Psychiatry and pain. In H. Merskey, J.D. Loesser, and R. Dubner (Eds.) *The paths of pain: 1975–2005.* Seattle, Washington: IASP Press.

Merskey, H., Loeser, J.D. and Dubner, R. (Eds.; 2005). *The paths of pain: 1975–2005.* Seattle, Washington: IASP Press.

Millroy, S. (2001). Scare-mongering over "hillbilly heroin" deprives the rest of us. www.foxnews.com August 5, 2001.

Mitchell, S.W. (1872). *Injuries of nerves and their consequences.* Philadelphia, PA: Lippincott (cited in Jackson, 2002).

Mitchell, S.W. (1904). *Doctor and patient.* Philadelphia, PA: Lippincott (cited in Jackson, 2002).

Moyers, B. (1993). *Healing and the mind.* New York: Doubleday.

Nielson, W. (2000). The concept of pain. In *Chronic Pain Initiative: Report of the chronic pain expert panel.* Toronto, Ontario: Workplace Safety and Insurance Board.

Olin, R. (1996). *What is FMS/CFS???,* (Keynote Speech, Seattle Fibromyalgia Conference) *Fibromyalgia Network Journal,* July, 3–6.

Pellegrino, M.L. (1996). *Understanding post-traumatic fibromyalgia.* Columbus, Ohio: Anadem Publications.

Rausch, V. (1980). Cholecystectomy with self-hypnosis. *The American Journal of Clinical Hypnosis 22(3): 124–129.*

Report of the Commission on the Evaluation of Pain. (1986). United States Department of Health and Human Services (SSATUB) 64-031. Washington, DC: Government Printing Office. (cited in Vasudevan, 1992).

Smythe, H. and Moldofsky, H.A. (1977). Two contributions to understanding the 'fibrositis' syndrome. *Bulletin of Rheumatic Diseases 8: 928-931.*

Spiegel, D. (2006). Editorial: Wedding hypnosis to the radiology suite. *Pain 126:* 3–4.

Starlanyl, D. (2009). Personal communication.

Starlanyl, D. (1999). *The fibromyalgia advocate.* Oakland, California: New Harbinger Publications.

Starlanyl, D. and Copeland, M. (1996). Fibromyalgia and chronic myofascial pain: A survival manual. *Oakland, California: New Harbinger Publications*

Steiner, T. (2004). Lifting the burden: The global campaign against headache. *Lancet Neurology* 3(4): 204-205.

Sumpton, J.E. and Moulin, D.E. (2008). Fibromyalgia: Presentation and management with a focus on pharmacological treatment. *Pain Research & Management,* 13(6): 477-483.

Taylor, H. and Curran, N. M. (1985). *The Nuprin pain report.* New York: Lewis Harris.

Teasell, R. (2000). Pathophysiology of chronic pain disorders. In *Chronic Pain Initiative: Report of the chronic pain expert panel.* Toronto, Ontario: Workplace Safety and Insurance Board.

Thorson, K. (2008). I offered to write a newswletter. In Then and now: Looking back at living with FM. *Fibromyalgia Network Journal,* October 2008, 17-20.

Tough, P. (2008). The alchemy of OxyContin. *New York Times Magazine* September 14 (taken from www.nytimes.com).

Turk, D., and Melzack, R. (1992) *Handbook of pain assessment.* New York: Guilford Press.

Turk, D., and Melzack, R. (2001). *Handbook of pain assessment. Second Edition.* New York: Guilford Press.

Turk, D., and Melzack, R. (1992). The measurement of pain and the assessment of people experiencing pain. In D. Turk and R. Melzack (eds.) *Handbook of pain assessment.* New York: Guilford Press.

Turk, D. and Winter, F. (2006). *The pain survival guide.* Washington, DC: American Psychological Association.

Vasudevan, S.V. (1992). Impairment, disability and functional capacity assessment. In D. Turk and R. Melzack. *Handbook of pain assessment.* New York: Guilford Press.

Vierck Jr., C.J. (2006). Mechanisms underlying development of spatially distributed chronic pain (fibromyalgia). *Pain 124:* 242–263.

Von Koroff, M., Dworkin, S.G., LeResche, L. and Kruger, A. (1988). An epidemiologic comparison of pain complaints. *Pain* 32: 33-40.

Von Koroff, M. (1992). Epidemiologic and survey methods: Chronic pain assessment. In D. Turk and R. Melzack (eds.) *Handbook of pain assessment.* New York: Guilford Press.

Wall, P. (2000). *The science of suffering.* New York: Columbia University Press.

Wallis, B.J., Lord, S.M. and Bogduk, N. (1997). Resolution of psychological distress of whiplash patients following treatment by radio frequency neurotomy: A randomized, double-blind, placebo-controlled trial. *Pain 7:* 15–22.

Walters, C. and Havens R.A. (1993). *Hypnotherapy for health, harmony, and peak performance: Expanding goals for psychotherapy*. New York: Brunner/Mazel.

Michael R. MacDonald
Some History and Background

I have been interested in helping people for a long time. Even at a young age, ten I think, I saw a young boy on the playground spin off of a slide and hurt himself. I was visiting with my aunt and uncle in Prince Edward Island at the time. The young boy did not seem to have any parents nearby, so I asked my aunt to take him home to get help. We ended up taking him to the hospital. I remember that no one seemed to want to do anything to help this boy. I felt I needed to do something. We were able to help him, thankfully. It felt good.

My first exposure to psychology was in my starting year at the University of Toronto, Erindale College campus. I seem to connect more easily with psychology, than with chemistry, math or physics. In my later undergraduate years, I began to major in psychology and was very fortunate to work with Professor Lester Krames. I was able to join his laboratory and do some independent research work. By then, I was hooked.

My next very lucky break came when I was accepted into the Master's and Ph.D. programs in clinical psychology at the University of Western Ontario (London, Ontario Canada). Only a few students are accepted into this program each year. I felt very fortunate. An even bigger break came from my being set up to work with Professor Nicholas Kuiper. He was a young and talented researcher. I was full of energy and ideas. He allowed me to work together with him on many of his research projects; a rare opportunity for a young graduate student.

In my second year of graduate school. I met the love of my life. My biggest break of all. She had an office two doors down and was working toward her Ph.D. in child psychology. She is still the love of my life.

Six years of graduate school flew by. In 1985, I graduated with a doctorate (Ph.D.) in clinical psychology and went about looking for work. I had been doing some part-time work with Dr. Gail Golden in her private practice. She agreed to hire me on. She was and still is a true inspiration for me.

I was also fortunate to find work in the Chronic Pain Disability Program at St. Mary's Hospital in London. Dr. Barry Death, a physical medicine specialist, ran this amazing multidisciplinary inpatient program. We specialized in treating patients with the most disabling forms of chronic pain. Often family doctors and specialists would call and ask for help with patients who were desperate, overwhelmed and frequenting hospital emergency rooms for treatment. In the chronic pain program, patients with chronic pain would be admitted for a six-week program (8 hours a day) of intensive treatment by a whole team of professionals. I learned a tremendous amount about chronic pain, and disability from Dr. Death and from the many patients we treated.

These experiences provided the foundation for my work for the next 20 years and counting.

My wife and I moved on to form our own private practice with a special interest in the care of people with chronic pain and fibromyalgia. There are eight of us in our group now. Over 90% of our patients suffer from multiple sources of chronic pain. Their lives are limited by painful injuries, as well as by high levels of stress (caused by their pain). Additional layers of limitation come from the impact of loss and widespread disruption to almost all aspects of their day to day lives. These multiple limitations are so overwhelming that individuals are willing to come and see anyone for help – even a psychologist.

I love my job. I get to work closely with people from all walks of life. I get to learn about their work, their families, their passions, as well as their injuries. People limited by pain, always tell me that they want their life back. I listen carefully to this. It becomes one of the main things we work on, hour after hour. I am still learning and still helping. It is a privilege to be able to help in any way I can.

Ordering More Books

I hope you have enjoyed this book and hope it has made your life even a little bit easier.

If you or your family or friends would like to order this book, it is available from:

Michael Renford Books
655 Wellington Road South, Suite 401
London, Ontario, Canada N6C 4R4

Books can also be purchased directly from:
www.UnbelievablePainControl.com
www.renfordbooks.com

Please come and visit me at these Websites. I am always adding new information to help you with your chronic pain and fibromyalgia.

I am also working on a new book to be called:
Unbelievably Real

This book is about reclaiming your credibility, recovering from pain flare-ups and losses and achieving long-term pain control. It should be finished over the next year. When it is ready, I will announce it in the Websites, noted above.

Thank you.

Michael R. MacDonald